D0274494

Edited by
SIDNEY BENJAMIN
ALLAN HOUSE
PETER JENKINS

Liaison Psychiatry

Defining Needs and Planning Services

GASKELL

Gaskell is an imprint of the Royal College of Psychiatrists,
17 Belgrave Square, London SW1X 8PG

British Library Cataloguing-in-Publication Data
A catalogue record for this book is available from
the British Library.

ISBN 0-902241-69-9

Distributed in North America
by American Psychiatric Press, Inc.
ISBN 0-88048-632-5

The views presented in this book do not necessarily reflect
those of the Royal College of Psychiatrists, and the publishers
are not responsible for any error of omission or fact.

The Royal College of Psychiatrists is a registered charity (no. 228636).

Printed by Bell & Bain Ltd., Glasgow.

Contents

List of contributors   vii
Introduction   ix

Part I. Planning liaison psychiatry services

1 Estimating needs and meeting demands
   Allan House and Gail Hodgson   3
2 The need for specialised services for chronic
   somatisers *Sidney Benjamin and Keith Bridges*   16
3 The need for specialist services for mood disorders
   in the medically ill *Peter Jenkins and Nahla Jamil* 24
4 The role of the nurse in consultation–liaison psychiatry
   Elaine Egan-Morriss, Richard Morriss and Allan House 34

Part II. Liaison psychiatry in practice

5 Setting up a consultation–liaison psychiatry service
   in South Gwent *Andrew Blewett and Peter Jenkins*   47
6 Liaison psychiatry in a large teaching hospital: the
   service at Leeds General Infirmary *Allan House*   58
7 Providing a psychiatric service to a large cancer
   hospital *Peter Maguire and Penelope Hopwood*   65
8 A child psychiatry liaison service
   Peter Loader   70
9 Liaison services for elderly people
   Susan Mary Benbow   76

Part III. Education and research in liaison psychiatry

10   Undergraduate teaching
     Gary Bell   95
11   Postgraduate training
     Elspeth Guthrie and Francis Creed   99
12   The relevance of research
     Elspeth Guthrie and Francis Creed   104

Appendix
Recommendations of the Liaison Group Executive
Committee for postgraduate training   114

Index   117

Contributors

Gary Bell, BA, MB, BS, MRCPsych, Consultant Psychiatrist, Royal National Orthopaedic Hospital, Stanmore, Middlesex HA7 4LP

Susan Mary Benbow, MSc, MRCPsych, Consultant Old Age Psychiatrist, Manchester Royal Infirmary, Oxford Road, Manchester M13 9WL

Sidney Benjamin, MD, MPhil, FRCPsych, Senior Lecturer and Honorary Consultant Psychiatrist, Department of Psychiatry, Manchester Royal Infirmary, Oxford Road, Manchester M13 9WL

Andrew Blewett, MRCPsych, Consultant Psychiatrist, Kettering General Hospital, Rottwell Road, Kettering NN16 8UZ

Keith Bridges, MD, MSc, MRCPsych, Consultant Psychiatrist and Honorary Associate Lecturer, Manchester Royal Infirmary, Oxford Road, Manchester M13 9WL

Francis Creed, MD, FRCP, FRCPsych, Professor of Psychiatry, Manchester Royal Infirmary, Oxford Road, Manchester M13 9WL

Elaine Egan-Morriss, RGN, RMN, DipHSM, Project Nurse in Resource Management and Information Technology, Royal Oldham Hospital, Oldham OL1 2JH

Elspeth Guthrie, MD, MRCPsych, Lecturer, Department of Psychiatry, Manchester Royal Infirmary, Oxford Road, Manchester M13 9WL

Gail Hodgson, PhD, MRCPsych, Consultant Psychiatrist, Coney Hill Hospital, Gloucester GL4 7QJ

Penelope Hopwood, MSc, MRCPsych, Senior Research Fellow, CRC Psychological Medicine Group, Stanley House, Christie Hospital, Manchester M20 9BX

Allan House, DM, MRCP, MRCPsych, Consultant Liaison Psychiatrist and Senior Lecturer, Leeds General Infirmary, Great George Street, Leeds LS1 3EX

Nahla Jamil, MRCP, MRCPsych, Consultant Psychiatrist, East Glamorgan Hospital, Church Village, Mid Glamorgan CF38 1AB

Peter Jenkins, MRCPsych, Consultant Liaison Psychiatrist, St Cadoc's Hospital, Newport, Gwent NP6 1XQ

Peter Loader, MRCPsych, Senior Lecturer and Honorary Consultant Child Psychiatrist, St Thomas' and Guy's Hospitals, and West Lambeth Community Care Trust, 35 Black Prince Road, London SE11 6JJ

Peter Maguire, BA, MBBChir, FRCPsych, Senior Lecturer and Honorary Consultant Psychiatrist, CRC Psychological Medicine Group, Stanley House, Christie Hospital, Manchester M20 9BX

Richard Morriss, MD, MMedSci, MRCPsych, Senior Lecturer and Honorary Consultant, Academic Unit of Psychiatry, Royal Preston Hospital, Preston, Lancashire PR2 4HT

Introduction

The provision of organised psychiatric services to other departments of general hospitals began in the United States of America in the 1920s and has developed rapidly since then. In the United Kingdom such services were almost unknown until the 1950s, and subsequent growth has been slow.

The extent of the need for general hospital psychiatric services, and the specialist knowledge and skills involved in providing them, have led to the creation of a few consultant posts in consultation–liaison psychiatry, but in most health districts services remain unplanned and unmanaged. The extent of service needs and provision is unmeasured; patients are assessed and treated by consultants who have not received specialised training in liaison work. There are few consultants who can give postgraduate trainees the comprehensive supervised experience that will enable them to provide better services for the future.

There is a wealth of evidence of the need for liaison psychiatry services. Patients in general hospitals have rates of psychiatric disorder substantially higher than those encountered in the community, and there are a number of reasons why these mental health needs should be met within the general hospital. Firstly, the problem may be so acute that delay occasioned by referral to an outside agency is unacceptable; examples include parasuicide assessment, crises on medical wards or presentations in the accident and emergency department. Secondly, chronic physical illness (particularly if its treatment is specialised) may take the patient to hospital so frequently that provision of psychiatric help away from the hospital is neither convenient nor feasible from the patient's point of view. Thirdly, there are cases where psychiatric disorder is so intimately tied up with presentation to the general hospital that failure to provide psychiatry on site effectively precludes the meeting of mental health needs at all; examples include psychiatric complications of severe physical illness, and the majority of severe somatising presentations.

Evidence of need for liaison services is matched by evidence of demand for them. Where such services have been introduced they have been accompanied by a rapid increase in the rate of referral for psychiatric assessment from medical and surgical specialities.

Nevertheless, we know from surveys undertaken in the UK and from our personal experience that actual provision of liaison services is extremely variable, patchy and at times non-existent. At the same time (and perhaps inevitably as a consequence) training opportunities in liaison psychiatry are limited. The result is that, while psychiatric work in general hospitals does (and must) go on, the service is often provided in a haphazard way which is neither satisfactory to its providers nor greatly appreciated by its recipients. Liaison services are rarely planned and delivered as a specific enterprise, but rather they are fitted into the pattern of general psychiatric service provision.

This unsatisfactory state of affairs has been recognised for some time in the UK. Why has it not improved? Part of the problem is a structural/organisational one, which in our opinion is at least as important as the problem of chronic under-resourcing which afflicts all areas of the NHS. Management structures and medical representative structures (which increasingly mirror each other) rarely allow any place for the representation of liaison psychiatry. Even within the Royal College of Psychiatrists, liaison psychiatry is officially seen as a part of general psychiatry. The result is that existing disorganisation simply replicates itself. One example is a historical lack of acknowledgement of specific manpower requirements in liaison psychiatry. Around the country consultant psychiatrists are being appointed to posts in general psychiatry with a small sessional commitment to liaison work, in which the liaison component is competing with general psychiatric commitments for time and limited resources. If appointed consultants have little training or experience in an established liaison service (as is usually the case), then they have no clear template from which to design the liaison component of their work. It is not surprising that we hear so often from such consultants that they would be keen to practise more liaison psychiatry if only they knew how to find the time and meet their other commitments.

It is a main objective of the Liaison Psychiatry Special Interest Group of the Royal College of Psychiatrists to change this state of affairs. With a relatively small number of senior practitioners in the field, the group has a large and predominantly young member-ship which actively supports regular conferences, workshops, and our biannual residential conference. In recent years we have contributed to joint clinical conferences with non-psychiatric colleagues in neurology, diabetes, cardiology and a range of other specialities. This publication arises as another initiative of the liaison group. We hope it will serve to summarise some of the discussions which we have held at our conferences and workshops, and give some flavour of our deliberations on the important topic of planning and developing liaison services in the UK.

The book is divided into three main sections. In the first we outline something of the scope of liaison services, the needs they should be designed to meet and the demands which will be placed upon them. Two specific clinical topics (chronic somatisation and mood disorder in the physically ill) are discussed to show that there are specialised clinical skills as well as organisational issues raised in considering liaison services. Whereas the management of mood disorders will (or should) usually be provided by liaison psychiatry services in all health districts, chronic somatisers present an example of a group that will sometimes require more specialised services, which cannot reasonably be provided in each district. Such services may be organised at a regional level, or for several adjacent districts. These issues are examined in Chapters 2 and 3.

Although multidisciplinary teams were originally regarded as essential to liaison psychiatry, we know of relatively few examples of services organised in this way in the UK. Chapter 4 examines the contribution that can be made by nurses. As in other parts of this book, we make no attempt to be comprehensive. We are aware that valuable contributions are made to liaison services by clinical psychologists, social workers and occupational therapists but, except in a few specific areas (such as social work involvement in the management of deliberate self-harm), their contribution in the UK does not appear to have been systematically studied.

In the second section, services are described, one in a district general hospital, and another in a teaching hospital, which indicate something about specific ways to deliver these clinical skills. The description of a psychiatric service to a regional cancer hospital illustrates the way that a service is organised for patients with a relatively common group of disorders, based initially on their presence at a specialised treatment site. Unusually, this service developed particularly as a consequence of research which demonstrated the skills of its staff and their clinical efficacy. The descriptions of services for children and for the elderly illustrate specific aspects of liaison psychiatry, and also the differences between models of consultation and liaison psychiatry and some of the ways in which they may develop.

From its inception, a major aim of liaison psychiatry was the education of medical students and internists about the psychosocial aspects of physical complaints, as distinct from psychiatrists teaching about mental illnesses. This has rarely been a feature of undergraduate psychiatric training in the United Kingdom. Similarly, postgraduate psychiatric training has provided few opportunities for acquiring the knowledge and skills required by liaison psychiatrists. Building for the future also requires that liaison psychiatry has a sound research base. The third section therefore discusses education, training and research.

This is not intended to be a comprehensive or exhaustive review of liaison psychiatry services. For example, we have not focused on the need for services in a number of particular areas such as deliberate self-harm, substance misuse, brain injury and confusional states. We have not discussed specific aspects of liaison services in the new NHS, such as contracting and budgeting. Instead we have approached general principles through worked examples.

By the same token we are not proposing a single blueprint or style of psychiatric services in the general hospital. For some, a consultation-based model will take precedence, while for others, formal specialist liaison work and joint clinical working will be more appropriate. Our aim throughout is to provoke and inform discussion rather than to prescribe.

We hope our deliberations will be of particular interest to three groups of people. First and foremost are service planners. This means *providers* in the mental illness units and general hospitals, and *purchasers*, both those in the health authorities and those general practice fund-holders whose patients will use general hospital services. Secondly, this book is relevant to all psychiatrists who spend time working in the general hospital, even when that work is not identified specifically as liaison psychiatry. Thirdly, we hope the book will be read by those psychiatrists in training who have an interest in this challenging and interesting area of work and will form the next generation of liaison psychiatrists.

We acknowledge the help of many colleagues, including members of the Executive of the Liaison Psychiatry Group of the Royal College of Psychiatrists. In particular, we are grateful to Dr Christopher Bass for his helpful and constructive comments.

Sidney Benjamin
Allan House
Peter Jenkins

Part I. Planning liaison psychiatry services

1 Estimating needs and meeting demands

ALLAN HOUSE and GAIL HODGSON

Where liaison psychiatry services exist in the UK, they are almost exclusively provided on a part-time basis. They may be provided by a National Health Service (NHS) general psychiatrist whose contract includes a sessional commitment to liaison work, or in a number of the larger teaching centres they are provided by consultants with academic appointments. There are only a handful of full-time NHS consultants whose major or sole clinical responsibility is for the provision of psychiatric services to the general hospital.

In a typical (non-teaching) health district, there is not likely to be a full-time liaison psychiatrist. Under such circumstances, how should liaison services be planned and provided? What is the need for a local liaison service, and what basic principles should guide decisions about the way in which the need is met? In particular, what is the minimum number of sessions in a consultant contract compatible with providing a viable liaison service, and how should the liaison work be allocated within those sessions?

These issues have been discussed on a number of occasions by the Liaison Psychiatry Group of the Royal College of Psychiatrists. For example, they were the focus of a workshop in Bristol and of workshops organised as part of the residential conference in liaison psychiatry held in York in 1991. This chapter outlines most of the content of the debate on this topic which has taken place within the liaison group and is based on the experience of its members. The first part takes the form of a review, while the second represents a worked example which may be of some practical value to those thinking about services in their own locality.

Estimating the need for liaison services

When planning a liaison psychiatry service, the first question we should ask is: what work will it be required to undertake?

In an ideal world, service planning would be based on epidemiological data from which a burden of need could be estimated. There are some such data which are of relevance. For example, we know the number of hospital attendances for deliberate self-harm, the rate of onset of mental illness after childbirth and the annual admission rates for head injuries or stroke.

Unfortunately, in other areas of extreme importance to liaison psychiatry our knowledge is less clear cut. For example, there is a large 'hidden' population of people with psychiatric problems who present to the health services with physical syndromes that are not based on physical pathology. Several reviews of neurological practice, gastroenterology and cardiology clinics have shown that somatic presentations like this may account for a quarter to a third of all new out-patient attendances. At the other end of the spectrum, the estimated prevalence of severe chronic somatising may be as high as 1% of the general population. In other words, we know that somatising is a common problem. What we do not know is the exact scale of the problem, or how many cases require management by a specialist liaison service.

By the same token there is general agreement that rates of psychiatric disorder among patients with severe physical illness are at least double those of the general population. Psychiatric problems may present as mood disturbance, or as disorders of adjustment characterised predominantly by behavioural problems such as poor compliance. These disorders have a considerable impact in the health service because they worsen the prognosis of physical illness and can increase lengths of stay in hospital, and perhaps increase physical morbidity and mortality. Again, however, we are not in a position to state exactly the need for psychiatric services to deal with them.

Estimating the demand for liaison services

An alternative approach to service planning is to estimate the demand for services, one indication of which is the use made of those facilities already in existence. Such an approach has the benefit of being more feasible in the short-term than planning led by need. The criticism that the demand for services may be unwarranted should, in future, be answered by medical audit. A cynic might also observe that if NHS services are to be determined by a process of bartering in the market place, then their provision will become increasingly demand-led rather than needs-based, so that demand-led service planning may be the more realistic approach for the future for reasons of political as well as empirical expediency.

There have been a number of published reports of work undertaken in UK liaison services. Members of the Liaison Psychiatry Group have also contributed unpublished figures from their own services to the discussion outlined here. What we know about demands in the UK for psychiatry in the general hospital is based on these types of sources. Largely informal as they are, these estimates of workload are reasonably consistent and at least indicate the approximate numbers of referrals likely to be encountered in a typical service.

Deliberate self-harm

Hospital attendances for deliberate self-harm have not declined substantially for a number of years. Rates remain at around 150–200 per 100 000 of the population, so that an average district with a population of about 250 000 will have 500 hospital attendances per year. The exact number of such cases which are referred for a psychiatric opinion depends on local referral policy, which has not been mandatory since the last Department of Health and Social Security guidelines (1984). It will also depend upon local policies about discharging patients directly from the accident and emergency department, rates for which vary from 15–50% of all hospital attendances.

Putting aside figures from Oxford and Edinburgh, which may not be typical because of their long-known research interests, psychiatric referral for deliberate self-harm runs at a rate of 100-150 per 100 000 per year in a number of services.

The arguments for having a liaison service to deal with these problems are:

(a) *Administrative efficiency and speed of response.* This is especially important if the liaison service is on-site while general psychiatrists have to travel in from elsewhere to see referrals.
(b) *Consistency of approach.* It is now more than a decade since Blake & Mitchell (1978) pointed out how widely general psychiatrists vary in the management decisions they make after parasuicide assessment. It is only by a coordinated centralised approach that such inconsistency can be

overcome. It is the rapid, efficient response and perceived rationality and consistency of management decisions which make dedicated parasuicide assessment services popular in the hospitals in which they exist.

(c) *Specific training and educational opportunities.* A liaison service dealing with deliberate self-harm provides training opportunities by focusing on a problem rather than treating it as an extra duty.

We have recently reviewed elsewhere the case for properly organised parasuicide services, which are logically best-placed in the general hospital (House *et al*, 1992).

Accident and emergency referrals

There are surprisingly few accounts of psychiatric disorders encountered in accident and emergency (A&E) departments. At Leeds General Infirmary, just under 2% of all A&E attendances leave with a primarily psychiatric diagnosis assigned by A&E staff. Excluding cases of deliberate self-harm, that amounts to just under 500 cases per year in one hospital, of whom about half are referred to a liaison psychiatrist or a liaison psychiatric nurse. In Nottingham, 150–200 referrals per year come from the A&E department (House & Jones, 1987), and Dunn & Fernando (1989) recently reported 121 referrals seen over a six-month period from one department. We know that this is only the tip of the iceberg.

How much of this work is true liaison depends on the local organisation of acute general psychiatry services. In a well-run sectorised service, the A&E department is not used as a clearing house for all acute mental illness, and unplanned contacts are predominantly for panic, somatisation, or drink or drug misuse.

Other ward referrals

In Nottingham, 10% of all new referrals to the psychiatric services came from the general hospitals once a liaison service was established; that amounted to 450–500 new contacts a year (House & Jones, 1987). From the Middlesex Hospital, Crisp (1968) reported 350 referrals per year, or about 4% of all medical admissions. In Leicester there were 300 referrals in the first 18 months of the establishment of a liaison service (Thomas, 1983). At Leeds General Infirmary there are about 300 ward referrals per year.

Many ward referrals are for one-off opinions, or only need follow-up while in hospital; a typical example would be referral for help with a confusional state. A small proportion are referred on to other parts of the psychiatric services. The proportion of ward contacts followed up in the liaison psychiatry clinic will depend on local policy and resources available, but will usually be about 40–50% of new contacts from ward referrals.

Out-patient contacts

Nearly all established liaison services run specialised out-patient clinics, which take referrals only from the general hospital. These may be used for new cases referred from non-psychiatric clinics in the hospital, or for the follow-up of cases already seen on the wards or in the A&E department by the liaison service.

At Leeds General Infirmary and in Manchester, new out-patient contact rates are of the order of 150 per year. In less established services or where the referral process is different, referral rates may be half of that figure or less (Brown & Cooper, 1987).

The composite picture

It is difficult to quote referral figures as rates because of uncertainty about what the correct denominator should be: district population, average daily hospital in-patient populations, annual admission or discharge rates. In larger centres with specialist services, adjustment will also have to be made for the effects upon psychiatric referral of case-mix in the medical population from which those referrals come.

TABLE 1.1
Predicted annual referral rates from a district general hospital
of 600 beds serving a population of 250 000,
once a liaison service is established

Source of referral	Annual rate
Deliberate self-harm	500
A&E episodes	150
Ward referrals	150
Out-patient contacts	
new	50–100
follow-up	500
Specialised liaison contacts	?

Nonetheless, using figures obtained from both published and unpublished reports, it is possible to estimate the likely total referral rates for liaison psychiatry services from a 'typical' district general hospital, with 500–600 beds serving a population of 250 000. The figures obtained are outlined in Table 1.1. They can be no more than an approximation because they are sensitive to the type and size of the hospital and the availability and popularity of the liaison service.

Deciding on the style of service provision

There are many views on which characteristics are most important when priorities in service planning have to be set: a focus on specific types of need, a comprehensive accessible service, competent delivery of special treatments, and so on. The problem is that a liaison psychiatry service may have to meet competing needs and demands, each of which could legitimately be given priority after the application of these general principles. For example, is acute assessment on the wards or in A&E more or less important than a specialist service for chronic somatisers, or than a coherently planned parasuicide assessment service?

Several factors influence the final shape of a liaison service, other than the already-mentioned estimation of likely workload and the application of some general principles of good practice.

The resources of the liaison team

A minimal service may comprise no more than sessional medical time. Input from psychiatric nursing, psychiatric social work, occupational therapy and clinical psychology enlarges the range of options for clinical practice. Even so, the skill-mix within a team may be one of the determinants of service provision. For example, it requires considerable experience to integrate the various components of care into a programme for the rehabilitation of a severe chronic somatiser.

The organisation of other local psychiatric services

There are likely to be services already established for psychiatry of the elderly, substance misuse, and perhaps other more discrete problems such as eating disorders, sexual dysfunction and HIV-related disorders. Local circumstances will determine whether these services have direct links with the general hospital, or whether the liaison service is the first port-of-call for the referring agent.

The expectations of other professionals

There are two groups of professionals with a particular interest in liaison psychiatry: non-psychiatrists in the general hospital, and psychiatrists working outside the general hospital. Both groups need to have their opinions canvassed and expectations identified. At the same time, both groups may have unrealistic expectations which need to be modified. Non-psychiatrists usually want easier access to psychiatry than is available. By this they mean a quick response to referral, with the Byzantine determinants of psychiatric responsibility (age, catchment area) sorted out by the psychiatrist. They also want an efficient parasuicide assessment service. Psychiatrists generally want a service that deals with all referrals from the general hospital; that is, not just those from certain teams or with certain sorts of problem. It is the administrative efficiency of a liaison service that appeals. These expectations are ignored at one's peril, because a flourishing liaison service will not develop without the support of these major 'stakeholders'. On the other hand, neither group may be aware of other reasons to develop a liaison service. Psychiatry in the general hospital can improve care for the medical patient, and (perhaps more persuasively) reduce morbidity and costs (Mumford *et al*, 1984). Non-psychiatrists may not be aware that their most difficult patients can be helped by psychiatric referral, if their past experience has been with a conventional psychiatric service which deals poorly with somatisers and those with problems adjusting to illness. Psychiatrists may need reminding that there are pay-offs in training opportunities and public relations in having a well-run liaison psychiatry service.

A worked example

So far we have reviewed some of the needs and demands which are met by a liaison psychiatry service. They arise from three main sources: patients in the general hospital; non-psychiatrists working in the general hospital; and psychiatrists working outside the hospital. To some extent the burden of illness in the patient population can be expressed quantitatively; the needs and expectations of other professionals working inside and outside the general hospital may be better described qualitatively. None can be ignored if a successful liaison psychiatry service is to be planned.

We will now outline the requirements for a liaison service in an 'average' non-teaching district with a population of about 250 000 people, served by a general hospital with 600 beds. We have assumed that the service will be led by a consultant psychiatrist. We are not prescribing an ideal service, but outlining a minimum one. It is possible to allocate fewer resources to liaison work than we are recommending, but our contention is that the result will be a service which is inefficient or non-functioning.

Allocating time

We have a reasonable idea of the sorts of clinical work which a liaison psychiatry service might undertake. What part might a consultant psychiatrist play in that work?

Firstly, there is *direct clinical work.* This might involve face-to-face patient contact following a consultation, or so-called liaison work where the face-to-face contact is with other staff who themselves undertake the appropriate treatment. Secondly, there is *clinical supervision.* Here a consultant might arrange for regular meetings with trainees in psychiatry or workers in other disciplines who are themselves undertaking the work. Supervision could take place individually or in groups. Supervision meetings can be time-tabled and relatively predictable. Thirdly, there is *administrative* and *organisational* work. A consultant working on a limited sessional basis may be quite unable to provide some clinical services – say to the A&E department, or for parasuicide assessment. Instead, it might be more appropriate to arrange to act in an organisational capacity, meeting A&E department consultant staff, discussing policy in the division of psychiatry, and arranging the necessary education and training (but not supervision) for those staff undertaking the work.

In reality these approaches overlap. It is difficult to provide a purely administrative and organisational input without on occasion becoming involved in individual case discussions. Clinical supervision will inevitably lead on occasions to face-to-face contact where a senior opinion is needed, or to administrative input where an organisational problem rather than a clinical one has been identified.

We can draw a basic grid within which to plan a commitment to each of these types of work, in each of the clinical areas where a liaison psychiatrist might be employed. A provisional grid is shown in Table 1.2. The figures require some explanation.

Administration and organisation of a clinical service with the caseload of a deliberate self-harm or A&E service will involve at least one meeting per week with colleagues, plus the time involved in trouble-shooting the problems identified. The alternative is to

Table 1.2
*Estimated sessional requirements for liaison psychiatry in a district
general hospital of 600 beds serving a population of 250 000*

	Administration/ organisation	Clinical supervision	Direct clinical work
Deliberate self-harm	½–1	2	5–6
A&E	½–1	2	–
Ward referrals	–	1	1–2
'Out-patients'	–	–	1–2
Liaison	?	?	?

adopt a hands-off approach which is likely to be neither popular nor effective.

Clinical supervision is calculated on the basis of a single daily meeting of one hour's duration with the staff who are undertaking the assessments. A little extra time is allowed for occasional direct clinical contact and travelling. One session per week is allocated to supervision of psychiatric trainees seeing ward referrals.

Direct clinical work is the most problematic and usually the most unrealistically planned part of the service. A minimal estimate would be that one out-patient clinic per week would suffice, particularly if a consultant were undertaking it in collaboration with a reasonably-experienced psychiatric trainee. Estimating ward referrals at two to three per week, then a further clinical session would be needed.

No figures are quoted for direct clinical work in the A&E department, which is unfeasible for a consultant on a sessional basis, nor for administrative/organisational work on the wards or in the out-patient clinic since it seems an inappropriate way of providing a service.

Additional time not shown on the grid would need to be allocated for the training either of psychiatric staff working in the general hospital, or of other staff seeing psychiatric patients in the A&E department, on the medical wards or for parasuicide assessment.

Planning an unrealistic liaison service

It is quite common to encounter liaison services planned on the basis of a small number of consultant sessions (say two or three) per week. Using Table 1.2 as a reference, we will examine two possible options for providing such a service.

Option 1

Three sessions per week could be devoted to direct clinical work with in- and out-patients, seeing ward referrals, following them up on the wards where appropriate, and seeing new and follow-up out-patients in a closed specialist clinic. It would need to be borne in mind that the ward referrals could not be planned on a regular basis and certainly not managed on a once-weekly visit. Such a sessional commitment would leave the deliberate self-harm and A&E services to be organised by somebody else and the clinical supervision in those areas would be undertaken by somebody else.

This option is unpopular with non-psychiatrists. Unless there is an alternative arrangement for the deliberate self-harm service, then the appointment of the liaison post will not achieve one of its main aims, which is to relieve the other general psychiatrists of the burden of repeated and unpredictable journeying to the general hospital.

If a different consultant is designated for the deliberate self-harm and A&E services then this division of labour might be successful, but will involve a total of more than three liaison sessions per week. One would wonder how efficient it was to have two consultants each working a small number of sessions in the same hospital.

Option 2

A consultant who is to take sole responsibility for all the general hospital tasks will need to dedicate at least one session per week to the organisational and administrative issues involved in providing a deliberate self-harm and A&E assessment service. The problem then becomes how to constrain ward referral and out-patient work so that it can be undertaken in two clinical sessions per week. The answer is that it cannot be done without severely restricting the referral process, since two sessions per week is not enough to see even the minimally-predicted four new referrals per week, with the follow-up visits they generate. Again, the problem of clinical supervision in the deliberate self-harm and A&E services has not been tackled, so that work is still generated for the general psychiatric services.

Any such sessional working arrangements are unsatisfactory, and we know from colleagues appointed to such posts that they prove unworkable in reality. Ward referral and out-patient work becomes progressively squeezed by other commitments so that it is undertaken on a haphazard out-of-hours basis. As a result, referral rates decline and referral threshold is raised in a direct contradiction of the aims of establishing a liaison service. Dissatisfaction with the provision of emergency assessment and deliberate self-harm assessment is similarly likely to be reflected in a decline in referral rates to other parts of the service.

The conclusion must be that a *psychiatric service cannot be provided to a reasonably-sized general hospital by a consultant working substantially less than five clinical sessions per week.*

Planning a realistic liaison service

The justification for an estimate of five sessions of consultant time is that the district general hospital generates enough psychiatric work to be regarded as the equivalent of half a community-based geographical sector/catchment area. Large teaching hospitals and hospitals in large deprived urban areas may generate enough work to be regarded as the equivalent of a full psychiatric sector or even more. It should go without saying that any catchment area responsibility would need to be reduced *pro rata*. How might five sessions be spent? One possibility is outlined below.

Clinical supervision of deliberate self-harm service	2 sessions
Clinical work and supervision of ward referrals	1.5 sessions
A&E, administration and organisation	0.5 sessions
Out-patient clinic	1 session

If arrangements are to be made for the establishment of specialised liaison links or for the provision of any psychiatric training or education in the general hospital, then further sessional time will be required.

Assembling a team

It is now widely accepted in general psychiatry that adequate services cannot be provided by a consultant psychiatrist working alone. The idea of a general hospital representing a 'functional' sector serves as a reminder of the benefit of multi-disciplinary team work in this as in any other field. As with any team, skill-mix is more important than the professional background of individual members. Particularly useful are skills in interviewing and assessment and in short-term psychological therapies, such as cognitive–behavioural therapy, crisis management, problem-solving, family therapy and interpersonal therapy. People from different professional backgrounds bring their own particular approach to clinical teams. Psychiatric nursing skills are particularly valuable, for example in nurse–nurse liaison where a difficult patient has to be managed on a surgical or medical ward, or in the A&E department. Many services employ nurses as part of a parasuicide assessment team. Nurse behaviour therapists are an under-exploited resource in liaison work. Rehabilitation therapists (occupational therapists and physiotherapists) are of help with the chronically ill who are under-functioning because of psychopathology, and with the management of somatisers. Clinical psychology offers a different perspective from the psychiatric one, on more complex or atypical cases.

A basic liaison team to start up a service might therefore comprise:

> Five sessions per week of consultant psychiatry time
> One full-time equivalent senior house officer or registrar in psychiatry
> Two liaison psychiatry nurses, specialist (G) grade
> Half-time equivalent clinical psychologist
> Secretarial support funded at the personal assistant grade
> Receptionist, clerical and audit assistance

Sessional input from psychiatric social work and from occupational therapy would be desirable, but in many places would have to be negotiated *ad hoc*, rather than built into the team.

The team should have an administrative base in the general hospital, and a centralised system for accepting referrals and making contact with others in the general hospital. Out-patient clinic space should be in the general hospital, in order to facilitate liaison with other medical specialities. It would also improve patients' attendance and compliance, because this environment is more familiar, and will help to reduce any perception of stigma in seeing a psychiatrist.

There is a consensus within the Liaison Group over these recommendations, coupled with a realisation that there are few hospitals which have the benefit of even this minimal service. Practical experience in liaison psychiatry supports the observation repeatedly heard from colleagues that a service provided at a lower level is not satisfying to work in and does not satisfy those for whom it is provided.

References

BLAKE, D. & MITCHELL, J. R. (1978) Self-poisoning: management of patients in Nottingham, 1976. *British Medical Journal,* 1032–1035.

BROWN, A. & COOPER, A. F. (1987) The impact of a liaison psychiatry service on patterns of referral in a general hospital. *British Journal of Psychiatry,* **150,** 83–87.

CRISP, A. H. (1968) The role of the psychiatrist in the general hospital. *Postgraduate Medical Journal,* **44,** 267–276.

DEPARTMENT OF HEALTH AND SOCIAL SECURITY (1984) The management of deliberate self-harm. *Health Notice* (84), 25. London: DHSS.

DUNN, J. & FERNANDO, R. (1989) Psychiatric presentations to an accident and emergency department. *Psychiatric Bulletin,* **13,** 672–674.

HOUSE, A. & JONES, S. (1987) The effects of establishing a psychiatric consultation-liaison service: changes in patterns of referral and care. *Health Trends,* **19,** 10–12.

——, OWENS, D. & STORER, D. (1992) Psychosocial intervention following attempted suicide: is there a case for better services? *International Review of Psychiatry,* **4,** 15–22.

MUMFORD, E., SCHLESINGER, H., GLASS, G., *et al* (1984), A new look at evidence about cost of medical utilization following mental health treatment. *American Journal of Psychiatry,* **141,** 1145–1158.

THOMAS, C. J. (1983) Referrals to a British liaison psychiatry service. *Health Trends,* **15,** 61–64.

Further reading

There is a series of papers in *General Hospital Psychiatry* (1987), vol. 9, concerning the marketing of consultation–liaison psychiatry:

PINCUS, H. A. Commentary, 347–349.

HOUPT, J. L. Products of consultation–liaison psychiatry, 350–353.

WISE, T. N. Segmenting and accessing the market in consultation–liaison psychiatry, 354-363.

HOLTZ, J. L. Communicating an effective message, 364–367.

STRAIN, J. J. Appraising market approaches for consultation–liaison psychiatry, 368–371.

2 The need for specialised services for chronic somatisers

SIDNEY BENJAMIN and KEITH BRIDGES

In the previous chapter, House & Hodgson refer to the important economic aspects of liaison psychiatry, especially concerning people with psychiatric problems who present with physical syndromes that are not based primarily on organic pathology. In hospitals these patients are mainly assessed and managed by medical and surgical specialities and this is likely to represent an ineffective and wasteful use of services. A recent study (Kroenke & Mangelsdorf, 1989) of common physical symptoms in 1000 out-patients in an internal medicine clinic found that an organic aetiology was clearly demonstrated for only 16% of symptoms, and that the cost of discovering organic pathology was high (over US$7000 per case of headache or back pain). Treatment was either not provided or was commonly ineffective for most symptoms.

The nature of the problem

In recent years, many medical presentations have been recognised as chronic forms of the phenomenon of somatisation, which has been defined as 'the expression of personal and social distress in an idiom of bodily complaints with medical help-seeking' (Kleinman & Kleinman, 1985). Somatisation is thought to be an important mechanism enabling people who are unsympathetic to mental disorders to benefit nonetheless from invalidism when they are psychologically distressed (Goldberg & Bridges, 1988). In chronic forms the physical complaints may be symptomatic of a chronic psychiatric disorder. Chronic symptoms may also occur when acute or sub-acute forms of somatisation persist, even after the treatment of an underlying mental disorder, so that bodily symptoms and preoccupation with physical illness remain salient, as a means of dealing with continuing life stresses. Iatrogenic factors may make an important contribution because of the differential reinforcement of physical symptoms (Bridges *et al*, 1991), which are then more likely to persist.

While somatisation can occur in any psychiatric illness, it is particularly common in depressive and anxiety disorders (Goldberg & Bridges, 1988), yet many of these illnesses are not detected by general practitioners. Some chronic forms have been regarded as representing the severe end of a continuum of somatisation and have been reified as a distinct nosological group known as the somatoform disorders (American Psychiatric Association, 1987). These include conversion disorder, hypochondriasis, somatoform pain disorder and somatisation disorder (previously known as Briquet's syndrome). The somatoform disorders are characterised by abnormal illness behaviour (Pilowsky, 1986), with physical complaints and severe physical and social disabilities which appear to be disproportionate to any evidence of organic disease (Bass & Murphy, 1991). The most severely disabled patients are chair- or bed-bound, and their families provide virtually all physical aspects of care. Other features include an excessive use of medical services for physical complaints (Zoccolillo & Cloninger, 1986), failure to be reassured by negative findings, 'doctor shopping', reluctance to recognise the relevance of psychological factors, and mutual hostility between patients and their doctors. These patients present a financial burden on health and social services, a loss to industry, and dependence on invalidity benefits for long periods (Bass & Murphy, 1991). Like those with sub-acute forms, a substantial proportion of these patients may not receive a psychiatric diagnosis either by physicians or psychiatrists. Consequently they are disadvantaged by not being offered more appropriate interventions.

Estimating needs

House & Hodgson (Chapter 1) rightly point to the difficulties inherent in assessing the extent of the need of this group. The patients believe that they have a physical and not a psychological problem, relatively few psychiatrists have been trained in the special skills required for assessment and formulation of management plans, and patients are unlikely to be referred unless services are available for diagnosis and treatment. Where services are lacking, these disorders are unlikely to be diagnosed, the patients receive unnecessary and often costly physical investigations and treatments, and the need for specialised psychiatric services remains unrecognised (Zoccolillo & Cloninger, 1986; Stern *et al*, 1993).

However, data are available that provide some indication of the prevalence, severity and effects of chronic somatisation. Epidemiological data have been reported on sub-acute forms of somatisation (Bridges & Goldberg, 1985) but the prevalence and inception rates of chronic disorders are not clear. Assessments in different medical settings are likely to be influenced by the choice of criteria for case definition and detection, and few studies have differentiated between acute and chronic disorders. We are unaware of any epidemiological study concerned with the development of chronicity. However, in the general population, data from the North American Epidemiologic Catchment Area (ECA) Program suggests a life-time prevalence for somatisation disorder (chronic by definition) of between 0.1% and 0.4% (Swartz *et al*, 1986). The methods used in this survey are likely to result in underassessment because they exclude many people who have features of somatisation but do not satisfy all the criteria for somatisation disorder. Applying alternative criteria to the same survey, the community-based prevalence for chronic or recurrent somatisation is likely to be 5–11.6% (these issues are summarised by Smith, 1991).

Thus a health district with a population of 250 000 will contain at least 250 residents with the most severe and chronic disorders. As many as 25 000 are likely to have recurrent or persistent problems of somatisation.

There is also evidence of somatisation in a broad range of medical and surgical settings (Zoccolillo & Cloninger, 1986; de Leon *et al*, 1987). Of a consecutive series of patients referred to a psychiatric liaison service from other hospital departments, de Leon *et al* (1987) found that nearly half were somatisers and 15% had somatoform disorders. Katon *et al* (1984) found that 48% of somatisers had a depressive illness and 33% had a somatoform disorder. Between 50% and 95% of patients seen in pain clinics have diagnosable psychiatric disorders (Benjamin *et al*, 1988), yet few in the UK are likely to see psychiatrists or clinical psychologists (Broome & Korshidian, 1982). Patients seen in this setting commonly present with somatoform disorders (Reich *et al*, 1983) and abnormal illness behaviour (Pilowsky, 1986). Many are a considerable burden on family and other carers (Flor *et al*, 1985; Bass & Murphy, 1991).

Thus the hospital-based data indicate that chronic somatising disorders are extremely common in this setting and support the evidence from community studies. In a well established hospital liaison service such as the one described in Leeds (House, Chapter

6) it is likely that there will be about 275 new ward and out-patient referrals each year who have a primary problem of somatisation. This is rather similar to our own experience in Manchester where one of us (SB) has seen approximately 150 newly referred chronic somatisers (mainly out-patients) each year and other consultants see at least as many (including more ward referrals) between them. Although such data provide some indication of the demand for services, for the reasons explained above they are likely to represent only a small proportion of the total need.

Meeting needs – the management of chronic somatisers

As with other mental disorders, only a minority of chronic somatisers are referred to psychiatrists. Some receive appropriate management in primary care or general medical settings. However, somatisers are often unrecognised by their doctors and consequently are not treated appropriately or referred to psychiatric services. In addition, these patients frequently fail to recognise the psychological distress from which their somatic symptoms arise; they are reluctant to see psychiatrists, and the process of referral calls for special skills (Bass & Benjamin, 1993). Psychiatric training based on mental hospital psychiatry (even when practised in a general hospital setting) rarely equips psychiatrists with the knowledge or skills required for the assessment and treatment of these patients (Creed & Guthrie, 1993). Thus those who are referred are often sent back to physicians with the opinion that there is no psychiatric disorder, together with inappropriate suggestions for further physical investigations.

It is likely that the majority of people with somatoform disorders are managed mainly in primary care, although the description by general practitioners of these 'heart-sink' patients indicates the difficult task that confronts them. The optimal form of management in this setting has yet to be evaluated, but some important principles are well recognised (Bass & Benjamin, 1993). These include: recognition of the disorder; containment rather than cure using regular scheduled appointments; one physician taking charge to ensure a consistent approach; close liaison with all doctors involved to limit unnecessary investigations and treatments; clear information given to patients and their families about the lack of physical pathology; explanations about the links between stress and the experience of physical symptoms; identifying and trying to resolve current psychosocial problems; and avoiding the suggestion that "nothing is wrong" (the patient knows something is) or that "it's all in the mind" (she knows that her body hurts) as this only leads to disbelief and mutual hostility.

The need for specialist services

Specific forms of intervention, when provided by those with specialist skills and expertise in their use, have been shown to bring about improvement for the majority of these patients. These include psychological approaches based on psychodynamic, behavioural and cognitive models. Antidepressants can sometimes contribute to the treatment of those with depressive disorders, anxiety-related symptoms or chronic pain, even in the absence of a mood disorder.

It is usually possible to engage some of these patients in psychiatric out-patient treatment, but others are unwilling to attend as they see their problems as physical. Out-patient care may be inadequate for the most severely disabled, but many are unwilling to be admitted as in-patients to a general psychiatric ward. Admission to the psychiatric ward is in any case unsatisfactory because the staff are unlikely to have the skills or the time required by these 'difficult' patients, when also trying to meet the needs of those with acute psychoses. Despite these limitations, some patients can be treated successfully in this setting (Kincey & Benjamin, 1984). Recently, the movement of resources from hospital to community care, the reductions in beds and in the total resources for psychiatry have led to the closure of such a service in Manchester which had previously been available for many years.

A liaison psychiatry service which has a separate ward (described by House, Chapter 6) may be more successful in these respects, but will still only be able to offer a limited service. A few specialist centres for the management of chronic somatisation and abnormal illness behaviour have been described (Blackwell, 1981; Lipowski, 1988; Shorter *et al*, 1992). They are likely to be more acceptable to patients because they can avoid psychiatric labelling, although the focus is still on psychological management. They are also able to develop the special skills required by staff and to provide the structure and consistency which is a key feature of effective treatment.

Pain clinics, which developed in the 1960s in the USA, present, at their best, a model for the specialised multidisciplinary management of chronic somatising patients who often suffer from complex interactions of mental and physical disorders (Benjamin *et al*,

1988). Assessment often involves psychiatrists and/or clinical psychologists, together with anaesthetists, neurologists, orthopaedic surgeons, nurses, occupational therapists, physiotherapists and social workers (Hallett & Pilowsky, 1982). For many patients this will lead to an out-patient or in-patient rehabilitation programme using some of the psychological methods referred to above. Recent reviews of outcome studies suggest that there is evidence for the efficacy of psychological treatments of chronic pain (Benjamin, 1989) and somatisation (Bass & Benjamin, 1993), with persistent improvement in symptoms and disability, and subsequent reduction in the use of medical services.

Economic issues

Several authors have reported a reduction in the use of general medical services resulting from psychiatric intervention for patients with co-existing physical disorders, but there have been few such studies of chronic somatisers. However, a number of reports on patients with chronic pain and one on somatisation disorder have concluded that, with specialised forms of treatment, their inappropriate uptake of medical services can be reduced significantly (Smith *et al*, 1986; Simmons *et al*, 1988). In addition, pain clinic treatment can result in return to work by the majority of those treated, and the savings in sickness benefits and accident compensation is potentially much greater than the cost of treatment (Peters *et al*, 1992). Although these studies involve only "partial economic analyses" (Drummond *et al*, 1987) they maintain that redeployment of resources for these patients to specific rehabilitation services would not only result in clinical and social benefits to them and their families, but also a net gain of resources elsewhere in the health and social services.

The personal and public costs of these chronic and disabling illnesses are high and are likely to remain so unless specialised rehabilitation services are developed. As resources for health care are limited, more detailed economic appraisals of services for chronic somatisers are urgently required. Such studies, using techniques that can be applied to psychiatric services (Glass & Goldberg, 1977; McGrath & Bridges, 1989) would provide planners with a meaningful basis for making decisions about the deployment of resources for these people. This is particularly important in the current climate of resource management, quality assurance and contractual arrangements between primary care and specialist services. Unfortunately, in practice there is little encouragement for such assessments to be carried out. In their absence, chronic somatisers will continue to impose an inappropriate demand on non-psychiatric services and are unlikely to benefit from forms of intervention that are known to be effective.

References

AMERICAN PSYCHIATRIC ASSOCIATION (1987) *Diagnostic and Statistical Manual of Mental Disorders* (3rd edn, revised)(DSM–III–R). Washington, DC: American Psychiatric Association.

BASS, C. & MURPHY, M. (1991) Somatisation disorder in a British teaching hospital. *British Journal of Clinical Practice*, **45**, 237–244.

—— & BENJAMIN, S. (1993) The management of chronic somatisation. *British Journal of Psychiatry*, **162**, 472–480.

BENJAMIN, S. (1989) Psychological treatment of chronic pain: a selective review. *Journal of Psychosomatic Research*, **33**, 121–131.

——, BARNES, D., BERGER, S., *et al* (1988) The relationship of chronic pain, mental illness and organic disorders. *Pain*, **32**, 185–195.

BLACKWELL, B. (1981) Biofeedback in a comprehensive behavioural medicine programme. *Biofeedback and Self-Regulation*, **6**, 445–472.

BRIDGES, K. W. & GOLDBERG, D. P. (1985) Somatic presentations of DSM–III–R psychiatric disorders in primary care. *Journal of Psychosomatic Research*, **29**, 563–569.

——, ——, EVANS, B., *et al* (1991) Determinants of somatization in primary care. *Psychological Medicine*, **21**, 473–483.

BROOME, A. & KORSHIDIAN, C. (1982) Are clinical psychologists interested in chronic pain? *Bulletin of the British Psychological Society*, **35**, 418–420.

CREED, F. & GUTHRIE, E. (1993) Interview techniques for the somatising patient. *British Journal of Psychiatry*, **162**, 204–211.

DE LEON, J., SAIZ-RUIZ, J., CHINCHILLA, A., *et al* (1987) Why do some psychiatric patients somatize? *Acta Psychiatrica Scandinavica*, **76**, 203–209.

DRUMMOND, M. F., STODDART, G. L. & TORRANCE, G. W. (1987) *Methods for the Economic Evaluation of Health Care Programmes*. Oxford: Oxford University Press.

FLOR, H., TURK, D. C. & RUDY, T. E. (1985) Pain and families. II. Assessment and treatment. *Pain*, **21**, 67–76.

GLASS, N. J. & GOLDBERG, D. P. (1977) Cost-benefit analysis and the evaluation of psychiatric services. *Psychological Medicine*, **7**, 701–707.

GOLDBERG, D. & BRIDGES, K. (1988) Somatic presentation of psychiatric illness in primary care. *Journal of Psychosomatic Research*, **32**, 137–144.

HALLETT, E. C. & PILOWSKY, I. (1982) The response to treatment in a multidisciplinary pain clinic. *Pain*, **12**, 365–374.

KATON, W., RIES, R. K. & KLEINMAN, A. (1984) A prospective DSM–III study of 100 consecutive somatization patients. *Comprehensive Psychiatry*, **25**, 305–314.

KINCEY, J. & BENJAMIN, S. (1984) Desynchrony following the treatment of pain behaviour. *Behaviour Research and Therapy*, **22**, 85–86.

KLEINMAN, A. & KLEINMAN, J. (1985) The interconnections among culture, depressive experience and the meanings of pain. In *Culture and Depression* (eds M. Kleinman & B. Good). Berkeley: University of California Press.

KROENKE, K. & MANGELSDORF, D. (1989) Common symptoms in ambulatory care: incidence, evaluation, therapy and outcome. *American Journal of Medicine*, **86**, 262–266.

LIPOWSKI, Z. J. (1988) An in-patient programme for persistent somatizers. *Canadian Journal of Psychiatry*, **33**, 275–278.

McGRATH, G. & BRIDGES, K. (1989) Appraising costs and benefits in psychiatric practice. In *The European Handbook of Psychiatry and Mental Health* (ed. A. Seva). Zaragossa: University of Zaragossa.

PETERS, J., LARGE, R. G. & ELKIND, G. (1992) Follow-up results from a randomised control trial evaluating in- and out-patient pain management programmes. *Pain*, **50**, 41–50.

PILOWSKY, I. (1986) Abnormal illness behaviour (dysnosognosia). *Psychotherapy and Psychosomatics*, **46**, 76–84.

REICH, J., TUPIN, J. P. & ABRAMOWITZ, S. I. (1983) Psychiatric diagnosis of chronic pain patients. *American Journal of Psychiatry*, **140**, 1495–1498.

SHORTER, E., ABBEY, S. E., GILLIES, L. A., *et al* (1992) In-patient treatment of persistent somatization. *Psychosomatics*, **33**, 295–301.

SIMMONS, J. W., AVANT, W. S., DENSKI, J., *et al* (1988) Determining successful pain clinic treatment through validation of cost-effectiveness. *Spine*, **13**, 342–344.

SMITH, G. R. (1991) *Somatization Disorder in the Medical Setting*. Washington, DC: American Psychiatric Press.

——, MONSON, R. A. & RAY, D. C. (1986) Psychiatric consultation in somatization disorder. *New England Journal of Medicine*, **314**, 1407–1413.

STERN, J., MURPHY, M. & BASS, C. (1993) Attitudes of British psychiatrists to the diagnosis of somatization disorder: a questionnaire study. *British Journal of Psychiatry*, **162**, 463–466.

SWARTZ, M., BLAZER, D., GEORGE, L., *et al* (1986) Somatization disorder in a community population. *American Journal of Psychiatry*, **143**, 1403–1408.

ZOCCOLILLO, M. S. & CLONINGER, C. R. (1986) Excess medical care of women with somatization disorder. *Southern Medical Journal*, **79**, 532–535.

3 The need for specialist services for mood disorders in the medically ill

PETER JENKINS and NAHLA JAMIL

It is not difficult to understand the association between physical illness and depression. Some medical illnesses are potent psychological stressors that affect self-esteem, body image, and the capacity to work and maintain social, family and marital relationships. For example, a sense of loss is likely to occur in a previously fit individual who develops rheumatoid arthritis, which leaves him/her relatively immobilised and unable to carry out simple activities. In studies of medical patients with high rates of depressive illness, diseases such as arthritis, neurological disorders, chronic lung disease and heart disease emerge as especially strongly associated with psychiatric illness (Katon & Sullivan, 1990). Elderly patients are also especially at risk; physical illness is the most frequent precipitant for depression in geriatric patients.

In this chapter we discuss problems that confront the liaison psychiatrist in the detection, management and treatment of mood disorders in the medically ill.

How prevalent is mood disorder in the medically ill?

The North American Epidemiologic Catchment Area (ECA) study attempted to measure the prevalence of a wide variety of psychiatric disorders in the general population (Regier *et al*, 1984). The prevalence of affective disorders was estimated to be 9.5% (Robins *et al*, 1984), and 6.7% of these met criteria for DSM–III–R major depressive disorder. These precise rates conceal the difficulties of diagnosing depression accurately and meaningfully in medical patients. The cut-off points used to identify cases of depression on rating scales may differ between studies, which can lead to substantial differences, not only in the observed rate of depression, but also in the sensitivity and specificity of the measure. House (1988) has provided an interesting account of the theoretical issues involved.

Rodin & Voshart's (1986) review of depression in the medically ill described a number of studies with prevalence ranging from 5% to 45% depending on the methods of case ascertainment used. They concluded that about a third of medical in-patients reported mild or moderate symptoms of depression and up to a quarter suffered from a depressive syndrome. This rate is significantly higher than the community prevalence reported in the ECA study.

Hospital patients with different physical disorders show variations in the prevalence of depressive illness. Maguire *et al* (1974) demonstrated a prevalence of 11.7% for depression in medical in-patients, whereas in a prospective study with a similar methodology we reported a prevalence of only 7% in surgical in-patients (Jenkins *et al*, 1990). Prevalence varies with the severity of the physical illness; the more severely ill patients have a higher prevalence of depressive disorder (Stewart *et al*, 1965). Prevalence is also affected by the physical diagnosis of the patient, so that, for example, patients with cancer commonly present with depression and also have a higher prevalence of depressive disorders than patients attending a diabetic out-patient clinic (Greer, 1983).

Problems with detection

Despite the high prevalence of depression in medically ill patients, at least a third of medical in-patients with psychiatric symptoms are not recognised throughout admission. Problems in the recognition of depression by physicians and surgeons were described by Maguire & Faulkner (1988), who divided the topic into four areas. Firstly, some patients report psychiatric symptoms which are recognised and appropriately managed by the medical staff; secondly, some patients report depressive symptoms which are not recognised and as a result go untreated; thirdly, in some patients the medical staff recognise symptoms of depressive disorder (even though they are not reported by the patient) but no action is taken, possibly because of the stigma of mental illness or lack of awareness of effective treatment interventions; and fourthly, some patients do not report symptoms, which then go unrecognised.

Despite these difficulties, patients with depressive disorders form a substantial proportion of those referred to consultation–liaison psychiatrists. In our own area, 35% of referrals to the South Gwent Consultation–Liaison Psychiatry Service were diagnosed as suffering from ICD–10 affective disorders. Based on our experience, 0.8 patients per bed per year can be expected to be referred to an organised liaison psychiatry service for treatment of depression.

Screening instruments

It has been suggested that recognition of depression in medical in-patients might be improved by using screening techniques (Moffic & Paykel, 1975). Meakin (1992) concluded that treatment validation of case criteria is required to demonstrate that screening for depression in medical patients is worthwhile; that is, any screening method must be directly tested against treatment outcome. This reflects the fact that scores on screening tests often have not only a low positive predictive value, but also that the disorders detected by the instrument may not have longitudinal stability. Modern studies should certainly employ a second stage diagnostic interview such as the Present State Examination (Wing *et al*, 1974), the Diagnostic Interview Schedule (Robins *et al*, 1981) or the Composite International Diagnostic Interview (Wittchen *et al*, 1991) to ascertain diagnoses in a structured fashion. It is possible that the limited validity of case identification by screening methods has accounted for the negative findings of some psychological interventions with medical in-patients (Goldberg, 1992).

If screening methods were widely adopted, however, they would identify a larger number of patients than could conceivably be seen by most liaison psychiatry services. This suggests that there is an important role for the education of non-psychiatrists in the detection and management of these patients.

How does mood disorder in the medically ill present?

For clinical purposes, one of the most important problems is the interpretation of what appear to be depressive symptoms but which, in a person with physical illness, may represent a coincidental primary depressive disorder, a symptom of a medical disorder, an iatrogenic effect of treatment, or a reaction to the stress of physical illness or hospitalisation (Series, 1992). Fatigue, insomnia, anorexia and pain are common examples of such symptoms which can be very difficult to evaluate. Cavanagh (1983) confirmed that the presence of somatic symptoms was a poor predictor of depression in the medically ill. They found that affective–cognitive symptoms such as persistent dysphoria and anhedonia, loss of self-esteem, inappropriate guilt, and a sense of being punished were good discriminators, while vegetative–somatic symptoms such as mild psychomotor retardation or agitation, fatigue, disturbance of sleep, anorexia, and weight loss discriminated less well, unless they were severe, out of proportion to the medical illness, and related in time to the other symptoms of depression.

In another recent study, Hawton *et al* (1990) found that several symptoms provided good discrimination between depressed medical patients and non-depressed medical controls. Cases were identified using the GHQ 30 Questionnaire, followed by an interview with the Present State Examination. (Patients were included if the index of definition was greater than or equal to five.) Discriminant function analysis was used to compare the symptom profiles of the patients with and without affective disorder, and it revealed that depressed mood, morning depression and hopelessness were good discriminators.

TABLE 3.1
Endicott criteria for depression in the medically ill

---

*Fearful or depressed appearance

*Social withdrawal or decreased talkativeness

Psychomotor retardation or agitation

Depressed mood, subjective or observed

Marked diminished interest or pleasure in most activities, most of the day

*Brooding, self-pity, or pessimism

Feelings of worthlessness or excessive or inappropriate guilt

Recurrent thoughts of death or suicide

*Mood is non-reactive to environmental events

Five out of nine symptoms for at least two weeks

*These four symptoms replace: (a) significant weight loss or gain (>5% of body weight); (b) insomnia or hypersomnia; (c) fatigue or loss of memory; (d) diminished ability to think or concentrate, or indecisiveness. See Endicott (1984) for further discussion.

These two studies illustrate the *substitutive* approach to diagnosis, whereby symptoms satisfying criteria for the diagnosis of depression in psychiatric patients are substituted by other symptoms. Endicott (1984) developed this further, and proposed criteria for the diagnosis of depression in patients with cancer, substituting the four somatic symptoms defined in the DSM–III–R criteria (American Psychiatric Association, 1987) with four cognitive–affective symptoms (Table 3.1).

Other approaches to diagnosing depression in the medically ill have been: *inclusive,* suggesting that patients with a lower level of symptom severity should be included; *exclusive,* suggesting that patients with any medical disorder should not be included; and *aetiological,* as in organic affective disorder (Yates, 1991). Each of these approaches has its protagonists, but in day-to-day clinical practice we recommend the Endicott criteria.

The importance of mood disorder in the medically ill

The failure to diagnose depression in medically ill patients has a number of deleterious consequences. Depressed medically ill patients perceive themselves as more ill than non-depressed patients and, as a consequence, tend to be heavy users of health services. This occurs because the depression may lead to 'amplification' of the physical symptoms of the medical illness. Failure to recognise this process may lead the physician to suspect worsening of the physical illness, which could result in further unnecessary investigations and inappropriate treatment (Katon & Sullivan, 1990). An increase in functional disability is also a common accompaniment, especially as the effects of physical illness and depression on functional capacity are cumulative (Wells *et al*, 1989). Depression also decreases the patients' motivation to care adequately for their illness, and lower rates of adherence to treatment regimes have been reported in patients with coronary artery disease and depression. All these facts suggest that detection of mood disorder is very important in medically ill patients (Table 3.2).

Mayou *et al* (1988) and Hawton (1981) have investigated the outcome of patients with both medical and psychiatric disorders.

TABLE 3.2
Consequences of failure to diagnose depression in medically ill patients

1. Patient perceives him/herself to be more ill (leads to 2 and 3)
2. More frequent consultations with doctors
3. Unnecessary investigations and inappropriate treatment
4. Impaired self-care
5. Increase in functional disability
6. Possible increased mortality (?)

They revealed that patients with emotional disorder, as detected by the Present State Examination, suffered considerably more medical, psychiatric and social problems than did controls during the remainder of admission and subsequent care. Furthermore, patients with mood disorder on admission continued to make greater demands than controls on medical, social and psychiatric services during the year following admission. They also had double the mortality rate, although this did not reach statistical significance and may have been attributable to more serious medical conditions on admission.

Further evidence of increased mortality related to depression and medical illness has been reported. For example, Carney *et al* (1988) found that depression at the time of angiography was the best predictor of a major cardiac event, including myocardial infarction, coronary bypass surgery, and angioplasty, during the 12 months following the diagnostic procedure.

Treatment

The treatment includes physical, psychological and social components, and each will be described in turn.

Physical treatments

Patients who meet diagnostic criteria for DSM–III–R major depressive disorder might be expected to respond to treatment with antidepressants. Series (1992) has written an extensive review of the use of antidepressant medication in the medically ill, and he concludes that it is primarily the risks which should determine the choice of antidepressant, and these must be separately evaluated for each patient.

Double-blind, placebo-controlled studies of the use of tricyclic antidepressants have demonstrated the efficacy of these drugs compared with placebo in relieving depressive symptoms. The newer selective serotonin reuptake inhibitors have potential in the management of depressed medically ill patients. For example, it may be that primary care doctors will be less likely to under-treat depression if using a single standard dose of antidepressant, giving these drugs an advantage in this group of patients.

Although some have urged caution in the use of these drugs in first-line treatment (Song *et al*, 1993), others have suggested that evaluating the safety and efficacy of the newer antidepressants in the medically ill should be a priority for future research (Gregory *et al*, 1992).

Psychological treatments

The efficacy of cognitive therapy in depressed medical patients has been described by Scott (1989). Cognitive therapy seems to be as effective as antidepressant therapy in patients suffering from mild to moderate depression, but the utility of this treatment in the physically ill is limited by the lack of trained therapists.

Ambitious research programmes are underway to evaluate the use of cognitive therapy in patients with 'negative cognitive sets', which have been shown to be of important prognostic significance in patients with certain cancers. The results of these studies are eagerly awaited (Greer *et al*, 1992).

For those patients with prominent symptoms of anxiety, clear benefit has been shown from non-pharmacological interventions such as relaxation therapy, particularly with patients suffering from irritable bowel syndrome (Guthrie *et al*, 1991).

Social treatments

Some hospital patients regress in the face of the stress of their physical illness or hospitalisation. Failure to comply with medical treatment can lead to difficult management problems and this may impair rehabilitation and lead to negative attitudes among the medical staff. Depressive illness may lead to accentuation of personality traits, which may appear to the staff as frank personality disorder. Social problems can act as important maintaining factors in depressed in-patients with physical illness, and addressing these, for example with a problem-solving approach (Hawton & Kirk, 1989), may lead to a resolution of some of the symptoms.

What special management skills are required?

The liaison psychiatrist needs to know about 'high risk' medical conditions such as multiple sclerosis (Steganer *et al*, 1992) as well as the range of treatments that can be effective in these disorders. This knowledge should not be limited to pharmacological approaches alone, although familiarity with the use of anti-depressant drugs is an essential requirement. A comprehensive knowledge of the side-effects and drug interactions which may occur with antidepressant therapy is also mandatory (Series, 1992).

In addition, the liaison psychiatrist should be able to distinguish between adjustment disorders and more severe mood disorders, which may be very difficult in patients with physical illness. A knowledge of psychological treatments such as problem-solving therapy and cognitive behavioural therapy is also needed, and these can be used in conjunction with drug treatments.

An awareness of the sort of disease processes and hospital procedures that can provoke or maintain mood disorder in medical in-patients is essential. A number of factors can increase the risk, such as a previous history of depressive illness or the sudden recrudescence of a chronic condition. The diagnosis or recurrence of cancer, or the stress of surgery can be triggers, while some treatments, including cancer therapy, corticosteroids, and certain anti-hypertensive and antipsychotic drugs can actually cause depression. A knowledge of these factors will aid the liaison psychiatrist in his/her dealings with these patients and their medical managers.

Conclusions

Mood disorders are common in the medically ill, especially those who are treated in hospital settings. These disorders are often undetected and untreated, and may have an adverse effect on the outcome of the physical disorder. The presentation of mood disorder in medically ill patients may be atypical and unfamiliar to psychiatrists who lack specialist experience in liaison psychiatry. Treatment can be effective but requires not only special skills but also collaboration with those providing medical care. Physicians and surgeons require further help in identifying mood disorders in their patients.

The applicability of screening procedures needs to be carefully considered. In our own service we have recently advised one unit with whom we have a close liaison to enquire routinely about and refer patients who have a history of a previous psychiatric disorder. The place for screening using more sophisticated screening instruments is as yet unclear.

There is an urgent requirement for the development of diagnostic criteria which are valid and reliable in this patient group. At present the Endicott criteria are recommended (Table 3.1). The impact of depressive disorder on outcome for patients with different physical illnesses has already been demonstrated by Wells *et al* (1989), who found high rates of functional disability in patients with both depression and physical illness. Further studies need to

4   The role of the nurse in consultation–liaison psychiatry

ELAINE EGAN-MORRISS,

RICHARD MORRISS and ALLAN HOUSE

In North America, liaison nursing is considered a subspeciality of psychiatric nursing (Nelson & Schilke, 1976). In the UK it has developed only in a few centres, according to local needs and with no established pattern. In this chapter we review descriptions of the practice of psychiatric nursing in general hospital work. Using our own service as a case study, we discuss possibilities for a more organised development of the role of the consultation–liaison psychiatric nurse.

Styles of work in liaison psychiatry nursing

In 'consultation' work a member of the medical or surgical team refers to the psychiatric team (which may include a psychiatric nurse) for an opinion on diagnosis or management of psychological problems. In 'liaison' work there is a close link between the medical or surgical team and a psychiatric nurse, who attends ward rounds and case conferences, or works regularly on the general ward. Discussion of patients' needs and supervision/support of the medical or surgical team replaces direct consultation (Lipowski, 1974). This approach is more labour-intensive but is probably more effective in identifying the psychological needs of patients, staff and others such as patients' families (Stickney & Hall, 1981).
    Examples of the *consultation* approach include:

(a) a nurse providing an on-call service to other wards while working in 'orthodox' nursing on a general psychiatric unit (Davis & Nelson, 1981);

(b) a nurse working as a full member of a multidisciplinary liaison psychiatry team and seeing patients for consultation when they are referred to the team (Lipowski, 1981; Lipowski & Wolston, 1981; Stickney *et al*, 1981; Hicks, 1989).

Examples of *liaison* work include:

(a) a psychiatrically trained nurse working as a member of a specific speciality team – with rape victims, in the accident and emergency (A&E) department (Atha *et al*, 1989*a,b,c*), or in an oncology service (Tunsmore, 1989, 1990);

(b) an independent clinical nurse specialist practising within a general hospital but not attached to a specific team (Nelson & Schilke, 1976; Stickney & Hall, 1981).

In practice, these two styles of work are not separate. Liaison nearly always leads to an increase in referrals for consultation, and good consultation is always accompanied by discussion about management with the referrer. Since it is increasingly common in the UK to use the term 'liaison' psychiatry to refer to all these aspects of general hospital work, this convention will be adopted in the remainder of this chapter.

The liaison nurse – independent specialist or part of a team?

The importance of the nurse as part of a liaison psychiatry team was argued by Lipowski & Wolston (1981). In a further article, Lipowski (1981) proposed a division of labour between the liaison nurse and liaison psychiatrist. The former should take direct referrals from medical or surgical nurses. They deal with nursing problems related to psychiatric complications, and only if necessary is a referral made to the medical members of the liaison team. Hicks (1989) also endorsed the importance of nurse-to-nurse referrals and found that high-stress areas of nursing (cardiology, neurosurgery and haematology) referred a large number of patients to the nurse, although referrals to the psychiatrists were previously low. However, she found that about half of the cases referred to the liaison nurse were subsequently referred to the psychiatrists for joint consultation. On the other hand, Stickney & Hall (1981) found that liaison nurses were often asked for help with problems which would not normally be referred for psychiatric intervention.

On different grounds, Jackson (1969) argued for an independent liaison nurse working on medical or surgical wards, believing that the nurse needed to be identified with the nursing profession rather than the medical psychiatric unit. This liaison arrangement meets a number of needs for the psychiatric nurse:

(a) for an administrative structure to deal with nursing (as opposed to medical or psychiatric) issues;
(b) for familiarity with the hospital routine, general nursing policies and procedures;
(c) for frequent personal and informal contact with the general hospital staff, which facilitates referrals.

The skills required by the liaison psychiatric nurse

The liaison nurse provides psychiatric expertise to medical and surgical nursing staff, not only to improve patient care but to enhance general nurses' skills (Lipowski, 1981). The skills required are clinical and administrative, and specific abilities in both these areas are needed by the liaison nurse to enable her to develop or improve services in the general hospital.

Consultation skills

Firstly, the liaison nurse requires clinical consultation skills in interviewing and assessment, especially to identify normal and pathological responses to physical illness (Jackson, 1969; Stickney & Hall, 1981; Tunsmore, 1990). However, the liaison nurse is not a substitute psychiatrist. The assessment should be a nursing one, emphasising those areas of adjustment (like attitudes to treatment and illness behaviour) which affect care most directly.

Secondly, counselling skills are needed in areas specific to liaison practice. Examples include teaching problem-solving as a means of learning to cope with physical illness, and dealing with body image disturbances which arise as a response to physical illness (Jackson, 1969; Nelson & Schilke, 1976; Lipowski & Wolston, 1981; Tunsmore, 1990). General skills such as experience in bereavement counselling and supportive psychotherapy are also important.

Thirdly, psychological interventions such as behavioural or cognitive therapy need to be tailored for use in medical populations. The treatment of serious physical illness may impose limitations on the types of therapy which can be undertaken. Involvement with a family may sometimes be the most appropriate direct intervention. Again, the intervention may involve some form of therapy, or it may be primarily educational, giving information regarding the illness, treatment, or outcome.

Liaison skills

The nurse needs skills to handle liaison contact with general nurses, gained through formal teaching which takes place in seminars and lectures, or informal teaching during discussion of specific problems on the wards.

A more direct input may take place when conflicts between patient and nursing staff lead to management difficulties (Jackson, 1969; Nelson & Schilke, 1976; Stickney *et al*, 1981). The liaison nurse enhances communication between patient, family and nursing staff (Stickney & Hall, 1981; Tunsmore, 1990) or enables nursing staff to express their feelings about an intractable situation so that it is less intrusive in day-to-day care tasks. When professional conflicts arise over differences of opinion between nursing and medical staff, the liaison nurse may be best placed to support general nurses and explore ways of dealing with the dilemma.

The liaison nurse acts as a resource to the rest of the hospital. Non-medical approaches to clinical problems such as clubs, societies, community facilities and self-help groups can provide support and counselling for patients and their families. The liaison nurse can provide information, and help to integrate these facilities into the general nursing plan. A good example of the value of this coordinating role is in the care of patients with HIV/AIDS. There may be more than one medical team involved, as well as voluntary agencies and community staff, at a time when communication may be impaired by natural concerns about confidentiality.

The nursing process in liaison psychiatry

The nursing process is widely used throughout the nursing profession, providing a systematic approach to direct patient care. In liaison nursing the same model can be followed, although with some modifications, for example to encompass liaison work which does not involve direct patient contact (Caplan, 1970). In the liaison process there are three phases: *orientation, working* and *termination.*

Orientation includes an interview between the nurse and the other professional. Topics covered include a description of the problem as perceived by the other professional, the expected goals for the intervention, the estimated time for the project and the key personnel involved.

The *working phase* consists of the four stages of assessment, planning, implementation and evaluation. The liaison nurse's assessment involves the accumulation and classification of the available information. When this is completed the nurse and referrer should have reached an agreement on the identified problems. In the planning stage, interventions are proposed to solve the problems and goals are identified. The implementation of care is supervised by the liaison psychiatric nurse, but much or all of the intervention will be carried out by the other staff member. The evaluation phase involves both the liaison nurse and the other staff member in determining the extent to which the interventions have met the stated goals.

At *termination* the liaison nurse and consultee discuss the completion of care and plan how the other staff member might handle similar problems in the future. The liaison nurse should also evaluate their own performance with their supervisor (a nurse or other professional).

The liaison nurse should also evaluate his/her own performance in *supervision*, which may be provided by a senior nursing colleague, a clinical psychologist or a liaison psychiatrist. The importance of supervision cannot be overstated. The professional background of the supervisor is relevant only in as much as it matches the needs of the patient. As well as maintaining the quality of individual casework, supervision helps clarify the question of clinical responsibility for any decisions made and actions taken.

This view of the liaison process is similar to the more general description of process in 'Peplau's model of nursing' (Peplau, 1952).

Liaison psychiatric nursing at Leeds General Infirmary

Leeds General Infirmary (LGI) is a large teaching hospital with 950 beds providing a complete range of district services, as well as regional specialities, including renal medicine and neurosurgery. The department of liaison psychiatry provides the only on-site adult psychiatric service to the hospital. The department has developed over the last 12 years, from a small general psychiatry facility with a 16-bed in-patient unit, into a speciality service which now undertakes only liaison work. The department is multidisciplinary, with clinical psychology, occupational therapy, and psychiatric social work input as well as medical and nursing time. Two consultants in liaison psychiatry work in the department.

There are two nursing roles which have evolved in the department, where nurses are either based on the liaison psychiatry ward, or working as liaison/community nurses.

Nursing on the liaison psychiatry in-patient/day-patient unit

The ward has 16 places which are used to provide a mixed in-patient/day-patient facility. Admissions come from a variety of sources including referrals from general medicine and surgical wards, the A&E department, general practitioners (rarely), liaison psychiatry clinics and from other psychiatric teams in the city. The major problems admitted can be classified as: physically ill patients with psychological problems or psychiatric illness; patients who present repeatedly to the hospital for other reasons (e.g. hypochondriasis, eating disorders); patients with abnormal illness behaviour, chronic pain and other varieties of somatising; people admitted acutely from medical wards for short-term crisis care. Two typical case examples are as follows:

Case example 1
A 54-year-old woman was referred from the dermatology ward, where she was being treated for non-healing radiotherapy skin-burns. She was agitated, restless and tearful. There had been several arguments with staff about analgesia, during which she would become uncontrollably distressed about inadequate pain-relief – throwing things around and shouting. Opiates were not controlling her pain. There were (unsubstantiated) suggestions that she might be disturbing her dressings. She was transferred to the liaison psychiatry ward for a pain management programme which included non-drug approaches. Continuing care of her skin was integrated with sessions discussing the personal and family impact of her cancer and its treatment. Opiate withdrawal was successful, and eventually she was able to tolerate living at home until she received (successful) skin-grafting.

Case example 2
A 44-year-old man with epilepsy had been admitted three times in six weeks to the neurology department with seizures, unsteadiness and falls. Observation of the attacks led to a diagnosis of pseudoseizures and anxiety attacks. The neurology nurses found that his attacks were worsened by attention, but that ignoring him left them with no idea how to plan discharge – discussion of which always led to a reappearance of unsteadiness. He was transferred for a programme aimed at teaching him anxiety control techniques and treating secondary agoraphobia, while exploring the social circumstances underlying his presentation, in

a setting where he could obtain consistent non-contingent attention. Problems with personal relationships and sexuality were identified, and although they were not resolved by the admission, he gained confidence sufficiently to be discharged with follow-up by a community psychiatric nurse.

It is our policy that the nurses on the ward should be doubly-qualified; that is, a registered mental nurse (RMN) and a registered general nurse (RGN). Each of the nurses acts as a primary nurse for a number of patients. Patients are likely to have a number of different disciplines involved in their care, including physicians, surgeons, physiotherapists, occupational therapists, social workers and dieticians. Only some of these staff work within the department; the key nurse will speak with all staff involved and will also ascertain the patient's perception of the problems. The nurse will present this information with his or her own observations and assessment to the multidisciplinary team (consultant psychiatrists, junior psychiatrists, psychiatric social workers, liaison/community nurses, other ward-based nursing staff and psychiatric occupational therapist) in the weekly ward reviews. After discussion, short-term and long-term goals are decided and management planned. These are later discussed with the patient by the key nurse and specific care plans are drawn up using the nursing process.

Management may include counselling, behavioural therapy, family and group work, education and medication. The style of working is like that in other areas of psychiatric nursing, although the content of direct work with patients is different. An important skill is the establishment of a suitable ward milieu for the care of patients, some of whom are seriously physically ill or dying, some of whom are somatisers, and some of whom have predominantly emotional problems with relatively minor physical disorders.

Occasionally one of the experienced ward-based nurses will be asked by the psychiatric consultant to assess a general medical/surgical patient on her own or jointly with the consultant.

The liaison/community nurses

A liaison nurse who works in the A&E department helps to identify attenders with psychological problems or psychiatric illness. The nurse is available during office hours for emergency calls, or referrals for follow-up are made the next day. A large part of the referrals from the A&E department involves people who have committed self-harm or who threatened to do so (Atha, 1989).

Case example 3
A 28-year-old man presented every one or two weeks with medically trivial drug-overdoses. He had been seen by several duty psychiatrists who did not think he was mentally ill; in any case he did not keep follow-up appointments. The CPN arranged a regular appointment with him, and arranged a system whereby the nurse was contacted if he presented between times, rather than continuing with the futile round of assessments by psychiatrists who did not know him. Initial contacts were hit-and-miss, but eventually the man came to attend more than half the appointments and started confiding details of an abused and neglected upbringing. Episodes of self-harm were not eradicated, but reduced in frequency; staff in the A&E department were pleased to have a simple and consistent line to take with him.

This nurse acts as a community psychiatric nurse (CPN) with the psychiatrists and ward-based nurses, following up out-patients and discharges from the ward. This role is extremely valuable and often neglected in liaison services. It allows community follow-up of patients whose problems are not easily dealt with by the general psychiatry services, such as somatisers and those with chronic physical illness.

Two specialist liaison nurses have been trained in behavioural and cognitive–behavioural therapies and their application in the general hospital. These are new posts, but they are already attracting referral of a wide range of problems from around the hospital. The nurses take referrals directly from members of the general medical and nursing staff and from other members of the department of liaison psychiatry. Referrals to this service are extremely diverse. They include eating disorders which complicate medical conditions, panic attacks associated with hypochondriasis, atypical chest pain, and psychosexual problems.

The fourth nurse in the department works with staff in the genito-urinary department, helping with the care of patients with AIDS/HIV and psychiatric problems. The work includes making links with wards involved in the care of these patients as well as undertaking out-patient and community follow-up.

In addition, liaison nurses have been employed in research projects; for example, problem-solving in the management of repeated deliberate self-harm patients (Salkovskis *et al*, 1990).

The liaison/community nurses are all based in the department of liaison psychiatry even when, as with the HIV/AIDS nurse, their main workload comes from another clinical department. Clinical responsibility for referrals resides with the referring clinician and the nurse therapist. The consultants in liaison psychiatry take clinical responsibility only if the original referral is to them or for joint assessment, or if requested by the nurse therapists.

Developing the role of the liaison nurse

Styles of working are obviously a major determinant of the comprehensiveness and depth of coverage which liaison nursing is able to offer. At the LGI the service has not fully developed 'outreach' into other parts of the hospital by nurses with specialist liaison links. The exception is the recently established and specially funded HIV/AIDS nurse. Our situation can be compared with that in other services where liaison nurses are fully employed undertaking parasuicide assessments and out-patient follow-up of these same patients, with no hospital-based liaison function.

Can we 'mix' approaches to allow comprehensive cover, but develop more personal relationships with other departments? One approach we have considered is a 'link-nurse' scheme, which involves nurses spending sessional time on chosen surgical or medical wards. During this time they can establish relationships with trained staff and undertake informal teaching. We would expect most referrals to be for indirect patient care. The relationship is reciprocal; general nursing skills are polished, and we gain a better idea of the sorts of issues which trouble nurses in other parts of the hospital. On a rotational basis this scheme offers some hope for small numbers of psychiatric nurses to establish relationships in a large hospital. It may also be a suitable model for involvement of psychiatric nurses in liaison work when the service is provided on a sessional basis by a psychiatric team with a commitment outside the hospital.

> **Case example 4**
> A 32-year-old woman had surgery for intractable back pain, but her post-operative care was complicated. She would have noisy rows with doctors and nurses, accusing them of refusing to give her medication and falsifying the prescription chart. She would often refuse to engage in physiotherapy, while complaining about slow recovery. Other patients complained about the atmosphere created by these scenes, and by her habit of watching a portable television in bed until late at night. The patient refused transfer to the liaison psychiatry in-patient unit, and was too immobile for discharge. A liaison nursing attachment helped the surgical staff develop a consistent approach to her management, and to handle limit-setting and confrontations with less anger and guilt. As a result she was able to modify her demands considerably and relationships on the ward improved.

Our view is that the liaison nurse functions most effectively as part of a multidisciplinary liaison team. Otherwise there are dangers of isolation from colleagues with psychological and psychiatric skills, of a loss of sense of perspective since other psychiatric services are not encountered, and of a tendency to restrict objectives because of a lack of ready access to colleagues from related disciplines.

The psychiatric nurse needs to develop certain skills to fulfil the role of the liaison nurse. For example, a basic understanding of behaviour modification techniques may be necessary to help with abnormal illness behaviour, while helping with adjustment to illness needs to be informed by an understanding of family dynamics. Engaging the difficult somatiser or nursing a patient who is both seriously physically ill and mentally disordered are other examples. Some of these skills can be learned formally; hence our policy of double-qualification for ward nurses. Others need to be acquired during clinical work, and it is our opinion that this needs to be in a specialist unit. As services move into the community, it is hard to find the appropriate experience in general psychiatry.

We know too little about the way in which nurses from one background (psychiatry) can work with staff and patients in another department. We are working with the consultation model outlined above, but we should be looking constantly for new approaches.

General hospital consultants, junior doctors, nurses and managers do not always understand the role of the liaison nurse. Most are unfamiliar with research which shows the usefulness of liaison nursing in areas where formal psychiatric intervention is not usually requested. Traditional medical working practices in British hospitals tend to be opposed to nurse-to-nurse referrals. Developing a liaison nursing service therefore involves convincing managers of its usefulness and cost-effectiveness in the long term, and demonstrating to clinicians that liaison nurses can work in their service without being disruptive or interfering.

Conclusions

Liaison psychiatry in the UK is more medically-oriented than any other branch of psychiatric practice. When consultants are appointed with a sessional commitment to provide a liaison service (the usual model) consideration is rarely given to the multidisciplinary team required. As a result the role of the liaison psychiatric nurse in Britain has been neglected. We hope this chapter will stimulate debate on the potential contribution of liaison nursing and how it can develop.

References

ATHA, C. (1989) The role of the CPN with clients who deliberately harm themselves. In *Community Psychiatric Nursing: A Research Perspective* (ed. C. Brooker), pp. 1–21. London: Chapman & Hall.

——, SALKOVSKIS, P. & STORER, D. (1989*a*) Accident and emergency: more questions than answers. *Nursing Times*, **85**, 28–31.

——, —— & —— (1989*b*) Accident and emergency: defining the problem. *Nursing Times*, **85**, 50–53.

——, —— & —— (1989*c*) Accident and emergency: problem solving treatment. *Nursing Times*, **85**, 45–47.

CAPLAN, G. (1970) *The Theory and Practice of Mental Health Consultation*. New York: Basic Books.

DAVIS, D. S. & NELSON, J. K. N. (1981) Referrals to psychiatric liaison nurses. *General Hospital Psychiatry*, **2**, 41–45.

HICKS, S. (1989) The psychiatric nurse in liaison psychiatry. *Australian and New Zealand Journal of Psychiatry*, **23**, 89–96.

JACKSON, H. A. (1969) The psychiatric nurse as a mental health consultant in a general hospital. *Nursing Clinics of North America*, **4**, 527–540.

LIPOWSKI, Z. J. (1974) Consultation liaison psychiatry: an overview. *American Journal of Psychiatry*, **131**, 623–630.

—— (1981) Liaison psychiatry, liaison nursing and behavioural medicine. *Comprehensive Psychiatry*, **22**, 554–561.

—— & WOLSTON, E. J. (1981) Liaison psychiatry: referral patterns and their stability over time. *American Journal of Psychiatry*, **138**, 1608–1611.

NELSON, J. K. N. & SCHILKE, D. A. (1976) The evolution of psychiatric liaison nursing. *Perspectives of Psychiatric Care*, **14**, 60–65.

PEPLAU, H. (1952) *Interpersonal Relations in Nursing*. New York: Putnam.

SALKOVSKIS, P., ATHA, C. & STORER, D. (1990) Cognitive behavioural problem solving in the treatment of patients who repeatedly attempt suicide: a controlled trial. *British Journal of Psychiatry*, **157**, 871–876.

STICKNEY, S. & HALL, R. (1981) The role of the nurse on a consultation liaison team. *Psychosomatics*, **22**, 229–235.

——, MOIR, G. & GARDNER, E. R. (1981) Psychiatric nurse consultations: who calls and why. *Journal of Psychiatric Nursing and Mental Health Services*, **19**, 22–26.

TUNSMORE, R. (1989) Liaison psychiatric nursing in oncology. *Nursing Times*, **85**, 54–56.

—— (1990) Setting the pace. *Nursing Times*, **86**, 29–32.

Part II. Liaison psychiatry in practice

5 Setting up a consultation–liaison psychiatry service in South Gwent

ANDREW BLEWETT and PETER JENKINS

There is general recognition that the psychiatric service offered to general medical units in the UK suffers from a range of deficiencies (Creed, 1991). Despite this recognition, action to redress these deficiencies has been slow. A variety of reasons for this state of affairs have been advanced. Firstly, there are deficiencies in the theoretical base of consultation–liaison psychiatry (CLP). Secondly, there are institutional and professional difficulties involved in any kind of change which involves altered practice where new approaches may be required. Thirdly, a general lack of resources compounded by inadequate information on possible additional demand and a desire to focus upon established areas of practice complicates the picture (Creed, 1991).

In South Gwent, recent changes in the staffing and structure of the psychiatric services in adult general psychiatry permitted the appointment of a consultant with special responsibility for liaison work and the subsequent development of a structured CLP service. We believe that the service now in operation achieves many if not all of the goals set out by Mayou for the development of CLP in the UK (Mayou, 1991), as well as those set by the Royal College of Psychiatrists for training purposes (Royal College of Psychiatrists' Group for Liaison Psychiatry, 1988). This service has been accomplished by the redeployment of existing resources in a non-teaching hospital where issues faced might be similar to those in other district general hospitals (DGHs) throughout the country.

The situation in South Gwent

Medical services in South Gwent medical unit comprise a total of 1575 beds serving 275 000 people. The majority of these beds are situated in the Newport Hospitals (Royal Gwent and St Woolos), with some in County Hospital, Pontypool, and the regional burns and plastic surgery unit at St Lawrence's Hospital, Chepstow.

Before May 1990, psychiatric services to these hospitals were provided by the sector consultant during working hours and by the duty consultant outside these times. Deliberate self-harm (DSH) cases were evaluated by the duty consultant's junior. Such arrangements are common in the majority of non-teaching DGH sites. This system produced a low referral rate for non-DSH cases, and led to confusion amongst referring doctors. As no consultant had specific responsibility for the service, such work was seen as an onerous additional commitment, complicating busy on-call duties in traditional general adult psychiatry. Recruitment difficulties prompted the Division of Psychiatry to convert an existing post in general adult psychiatry to a post (now occupied by one of the authors (PLJ)) with a reduced sector catchment population (28 000) and with five sessions devoted to CLP. This appointment allowed a reassessment of the demand for psychiatric services within the DGH for mental health care, and led to the formulation of a strategy to meet these needs (Jenkins, 1991).

Aims of the consultation–liaison service

The mission of the CLP service was defined as follows: 'to improve patient care by providing psychiatric expertise to assist the hospital treatment team in their overall management of individual patients by consultation and, where appropriate, liaison with those teams'.

Consultation is defined as 'the psychiatrist acting to evaluate those patients who are identified as requiring psychiatric assessment and treatment by their treating physician or surgeon'.

Liaison is defined as 'the psychiatrist joining the treatment team of another discipline and cooperating with the team in the management of patients' psychiatric and psychological problems on a routine basis'.

Before starting the service, a questionnaire was sent to all consultants of the South Gwent unit. The purpose of this questionnaire was to assess attitudes and likely demand, and to enable goals to be set which met the expressed needs of the non-psychiatric consultants (Hanslip, 1991). The questionnaire also introduced the service and the new consultant, laying the ground for future educational and research collaboration. Following the analysis of responses, six goals were established for the CLP service (see Table 5.1).

TABLE 5.1
Goals of the consultation–liaison service

1. The consultation–liaison service will provide supervised assessment of all cases of deliberate self-harm within 24 hours of admission to the hospital.

2. The consultation–liaison service will offer a consultant/senior registrar-delivered service to all wards at the Newport Hospitals which will see all referred current in-patients within one working day of referral. (Emergency referrals within office hours will be dealt with by the consultation liaison service. After working hours the duty consultant should be contacted.)

3. The consultation–liaison service will offer an out-patient consultation service from the Liaison Psychiatry Clinic at the district general hospital.

4. The consultation–liaison service will offer a liaison service to the regional burns unit at Chepstow.

5. The consultation–liaison service will have an active educational role.

6. The consultation–liaison service will have an active research programme.

Goal achievements

Deliberate self-harm

The Royal Gwent Hospital has the benefit of a short-stay unit allowing the admission of DSH cases for overnight observation. There are approximately 800 cases of DSH admitted each year, 85% of whom are admitted to the short-stay unit, and 15% to other (medical) wards.

Since May 1990, consultant responsibility for the psychiatric assessment of cases of DSH has rested with one consultant (PLJ). During the week, assessments continue to be made by the on-call consultant's junior, and at weekends by the duty consultant or senior registrar. Initially no changes were made to the system whereby DSH cases were seen as well as the usual clinical commitments. The effect of single consultant responsibility was to enhance supervision of the juniors and allow the identification of problems in consultation with the staff of the short-stay unit. It also generated referrals to the newly designated CLP clinic at the DGH.

In order to clarify the issues involved in the DSH service, a detailed medical audit of cases was undertaken between 1 September and 1 December 1990 (Table 5.2).

TABLE 5.2
Deliberate self-harm assessments over three months, 1990

No. admitted	164	
No. assessed	121	(74%)
Of these:		
psychiatric intervention	34	(28%)
CLP clinic	7	(6%)
referred elsewhere	15	(12%)
admitted to psychiatry	12	(10%)
admitted to medicine	11	(9%)
offered no follow-up	54	(45%)
Quality of case records:		
description of circumstances	46	(35%)
any mental state	28	(21%)
suicidal intent/risk recorded	51	(39%)
follow-up specified	34	(26%)

(The quality of the information recorded in the accident and emergency (A&E) department notes was found to be very variable and this resulted in an educational effort directed at the junior doctors.)

A mean of 1.8 DSH cases were seen daily on the short-stay unit. Some complaints had been received that assessments were too late in the day. Thirty-six dates chosen at random were assessed and the timing of arrival of the psychiatrist noted. On eight (22%) occasions the psychiatrist arrived by 10 am, and on 18 by midday (49%). As medical discharge occurred before 9 am, the system allowing 29% of patients to wait over three hours for assessment was clearly unsatisfactory and may have contributed to the fact that only 74% of all cases were assessed. Another surprising finding was that 38% of those assessed were already in contact with the psychiatric services.

These figures make salutary reading, and when presented caused surprise at the poor level of service prevailing. Unfortunately, there is no reason to expect that services in other districts are better, and they may be worse (Hawton & Catalan, 1987). Whereas a good system was theoretically in place, medical audit clearly demonstrated deficiencies. The lack of information about the overdose, mental state, suicide risk and follow-up in those patients who were assessed made the notes unhelpful and allowed room for inadequate management.

The results of the audit led to a complete revision of this aspect of service provision. Currently, three designated juniors have responsibility on a rota basis which does not conflict with their other clinical commitments, allowing them to visit at 9 am daily. Weekend arrangements remain unchanged.

TABLE 5.3
Reasons for ward referrals to CLP service (n=69)

Current psychiatric symptoms	22
Suicide attempt	14
Substance abuse	12
Unexplained symptoms	11
Previous psychiatric history	11
Coping problems	9
Patient's judgement queried	3
Compliance problem	2
Patient request	2
Staff issue	2
Known to CLP service	1
Homicidal threats	1

CLP service to in-patients (ward referrals)

The service has been made available to all in-patient facilities in South Gwent. Initial planning included the circulation of detailed memos explaining clearly how referrals could be made directly to the CLP team by phone, with information on the proposed response. This included the goal of rapid assessment, and the format of written information passed back to the referrer.

During an initial six-month period, from 8 August 1990 to 8 February 1991, 69 referrals were made, at a mean rate of 11.5 per month (Table 5.3). Table 5.4 shows the principal somatic and psychiatric diagnoses. Of the 69 referrals, 47 were from the Newport Hospitals, 14 from St Lawrence Hospital, and 8 from other hospitals. Breakdown by speciality is shown in Table 5.5. Annual rates of referral by the major specialities are also shown. These can be seen as minimum likely rates for any equivalent DGH service.

TABLE 5.4
Somatic and psychiatric diagnoses of CLP referrals (n=69)

Somatic		Psychiatric	
Injury	15	Major depression	20
None	10	Substance abuse	8
Unknown	10	Adjustment disorders	7
Metabolic	6	Combined alcohol	5
Cancer	6	Psychoses	4
Cerebrovascular	5	Others	15
Self-inflicted	5	Not recorded	6
Endocrine	4	Not axis 1	4
Respiratory	2		
Haematological	1		
Benign neoplasm	1		

TABLE 5.5
Consultation–liaison referrals by speciality from the Newport hospitals (n=47)

	Rate		Rate per year per bed
Medicine	33	(77%)	0.26
Surgery	10	(21%)	0.04
ICU	2	(4%)	–
A&E	1	(2%)	–
Ob/gyn.	1	(2%)	–

Since February 1991 the service has participated in the European Consultation–Liaison Workgroup (ECLW) study, looking at all aspects of referral and psychiatric management and some aspects of outcome. This has provided a detailed data base for the 38 cases seen between 1 February and 30 April, 1991 (Table 5.6).

The goals of the service specify that ward referrals will be seen within one working day, and this was achieved 86% of the time. Most referrals originated from general medical services, which is to be expected as they have a higher prevalence of psychological morbidity than general surgical services (Maguire *et al*, 1974). A third of referred patients were already known to the psychiatric services, and 60% were offered some form of psychiatric follow-up. These figures do not include consultations requested from psycho-geriatric services (*n*=30) or child psychiatry service consultations (*n*=10).

TABLE 5.6
European Consultation–Liaison Workgroup: preliminary referral data[1] for South Gwent (1 February–30 April 1991)

Place		
Newport DGH	33	(87%)
other hospitals	5	(13%)
Known to psychiatric services	14	(37%)
Intervention data		
mean delay between referral and assessment	0.8 days	
seen within one day	33	(87%)
mean consultation time	51 mins	
followed up on ward	10	(26%)
CLP clinic follow-up	5	(13%)
other psychiatry service follow-up	18	(47%)
Source		
medicine	26	(68%)
surgery	7	(18%)
burns/plastic	3	(7%)
A&E	2	(5%)

1. For 19 men and 19 women (n=38), mean age = 49.5.

The liaison out-patient clinic

The weekly general psychiatric clinic at the Royal Gwent Hospital was refocused over the course of a year by discharging or reallocating general psychiatry patients, and seeing only new liaison out-patient referrals. The clinic accepts urgent referrals from the DSH assessment service, follow-up of ward referrals and out-patient referrals from consultants in the Newport and other hospitals. About 10% of referrals are extra-contractual.

After 2 May 1991, the availability of the clinic became more widely known and 24 patients were examined over a four-month period (Table 5.7). In common with the consultant's general psychiatry clinic, there is a policy to allow no patient to wait for more than four weeks, and all patients are given assigned appointment times. Both medical and psychiatric notes are available. There was a substantial increase in numbers referred. Again the majority of patients were referred by physicians. Several patients referred from obstetrics and gynaecology were pregnant patients who had had previous postnatal depressive illness and were followed up after in-patient admission for delivery.

TABLE 5.7
CLP clinic referrals[1] over four months

Source		
medicine	13	(54%)
ob/gyn.	4	(17%)
all surgery	7	(29%)
Reasons stated for referral		
depression	10	
alcohol	2	
PTSD	2	
conversion	2	
PFAPC	2	
coping	2	
epilepsy	1	
anorexia	1	
panic	1	
sexual	1	
Projected annualised activity		
referrals, other specialities	72	
DSH service referrals	28	
ward consults follow-up	20	
total	*120*	

1. For 8 men and 16 women (*n*=24), 65% under 45 years of age.

Liaison service to the regional burns unit

The burns unit based at St Lawrence's Hospital, Chepstow, was identified as an area of likely special need on the basis of previous literature (Welch, 1991). The unit has a ten-bed specialised burns ward, 25 associated beds and 102 beds for plastic surgery. Particular areas of concern included the management of delirium and substance abuse (Swenson, 1991). It was envisaged that psychological and educational input might later be required by the staff (Antebi & Ambler, 1989). Currently plans are in hand to audit the first 50 consultations requested and present these results to the plastic surgery division in order to plan service development.

One area where collaboration has already occurred has been in a ten-year retrospective study of self-inflicted burns conducted by registrars from psychiatry and plastic surgery. The child psychiatry service also offers a clinic within the unit every other week.

The recent Gulf War stimulated a useful period of collaboration based upon the existing referral mechanism. Arrangements were made for continuous availability of senior registrars in psychiatry and also for Arabic-speaking psychiatrists. Staff consultation and support were organised using a panel of trained counsellors from a variety of professional backgrounds. Thankfully these arrangements were not called into use, but they served to raise the profile of this area of need within the mental illness services.

Educational role

Training standards in CLP were recently considered by the Liaison Group of the Royal College of Psychiatrists (Royal College of Psychiatrists' Group for Liaison Psychiatry, 1988). In our service, regular monthly case conferences are held as part of the general professional training for junior doctors. The MSc in Clinical Psychiatry of the University of Wales' College of Medicine offers a seminar series in CLP. Links with nursing staff have been established and a variety of opportunities for involvement in the medical unit's educational programmes have been sought. Since April 1991 a senior registrar placement has been approved and the first senior registrar has been appointed (AB).

Research

Research offers a number of advantages. Firstly, it enables close cooperation between the CLP service and other groups such as surgeons; secondly, there is a deficiency of knowledge about many basic questions regarding the occurrence of psychological morbidity, and research enables limited resources to be focused in a manner which addresses these issues.

The South Gwent CLP service is one of eight UK centres participating in a multinational EEC-funded study of the effectiveness of mental health care delivery in DGH sites (Huyse, 1990). This study will offer a range of data about the backgrounds of the patients, their problems, what interventions are advised and how long intervention takes.

One study has been completed in the burns unit (Sonneborn & Vanstraelen, 1992). A collaborative study of intervention in severe treatment-resistant mastalgia is currently proceeding with the surgery division. A prospective study of irritable bowel syndrome is at an advanced stage. Research funding for studies of the effects of depression upon outcome and length of hospital stay has been sought to build upon the ECLW data.

Medical audit of CLP services

The volume of cases and the quality of service can be measured on a regular basis against the performance standards which have been laid down in the goals and objectives. This forms the basis for regular reports to the psychiatry division and the medical unit. In the instance described regarding the DSH service, the audit process led to a complete reorganisation of service provision. Audit is seen as an integral part of the CLP service, as it enhances the quality of care. In addition, it demonstrates how much activity is undertaken that is not reflected in the traditional volume descriptors of business and strategic plans, which tend to be based on traditional asylum psychiatry.

Conclusions

There is growing concern about the psychological care of patients in UK hospitals and evidence of deficiencies in the mental health care of these patients. A lack of commitment to CLP and institutional inertia play a part. Most CLP activity consists of assessing DSH cases and is seen as an onerous chore best left to inexperienced juniors. Ward referrals are handled on an emergency basis, leading to understandable frustration for both psychiatrists and other specialists who do not receive the service they deserve. The DGH is a place of high psychological morbidity, and failure to provide adequate management of psychiatric illness in the medically ill may adversely influence outcome and increase health care use.

The service described is an effective way of meeting the need for psychiatric services within the DGH. The increase in referral rates suggests that there is a large hidden morbidity of patients who do not receive necessary psychiatric assessment. Overcoming problems between psychiatrists and other medical groups requires a willingness on the part of psychiatrists to alter their traditional patterns of working, which usually reflect the requirements of the psychiatric institution and not the patient. Key areas include simplicity of referral to a named individual, rapidity of response and clarity of recommendations. Busy surgeons do not appreciate a lengthy discourse on psychodynamics when what is needed is explicit advice, nor do they need to be told that obviously disturbed people are "not ill" just because they do not have a psychotic disorder. Psychiatrists need to be familiar with the medical environment and modern medical and surgical treatments – a familiarity which is sometimes sadly lacking.

The establishment of additional services will, it is hoped, achieve a recognition of the patient as a whole and enable effective intervention at a psychological level. In the past, CLP has been seen as a marginal activity by both other consultants and psychiatrists themselves. A large DGH such as ours creates an additional demand for services equivalent to another 30 000–40 000 people in the area. There is an abundance of goodwill from the general hospital doctors who welcome constructive advice on the management issues they face. There is increasing awareness among psychiatrists that CLP is not the same as community psychiatry or general psychiatry, because the patient mix and the social environment are different from those referred from general practice or rehoused in community care projects. The process of meeting the needs of this patient population is well underway in South Gwent.

References

ANTEBI, D. & AMBLER, N. R. (1989) A staff support group in a burns unit: managing patients' psychological needs. *Psychiatric Bulletin*, **13**, 65–66.

CREED, F. (1991) Liaison psychiatry in the 21st century – a review. *Journal of the Royal Society of Medicine*, **8**, 414–417.

HANSLIP, J. M. (1991) Psychiatry in the district general hospital. The effects of a consultation–liaison psychiatry service on hospital doctors' attitudes and referral patterns. MMedSci thesis, University of Leeds Medical School.

HAWTON, K. & CATALAN, J. (1987) *Attempted Suicide. A Practical Guide to its Nature and Management* (2nd edn). Oxford: Oxford University Press.

HUYSE, F. (1990) The ECLW study: a short introduction. Amsterdam: Dept of Psychiatry, The Free University.

JENKINS, P. L. (1991) *The South Gwent Consultation Liaison Psychiatric Service.* Poster at The Royal College of Psychiatrists AGM, Brighton.

MAGUIRE, G. P., JULIER, D. L., HAWTON, K. E., *et al* (1974) Psychiatric referral and morbidity on two medical wards. *British Medical Journal*, **1**, 268–270.

MAYOU, R. (1991) What should British consultation–liaison psychiatry be doing? *General Hospital Psychiatry*, **13**, 261–266.

ROYAL COLLEGE OF PSYCHIATRISTS' GROUP FOR LIAISON PSYCHIATRY (1988) Guidelines for training in liaison psychiatry. *Psychiatric Bulletin*, **12**, 389–390.

SONNEBORN, C. K. & VANSTRAELEN, P. M. (1992) A retrospective study of self-inflicted burns. *General Hospital Psychiatry*, **14**, 404–407.

SWENSON, J. R. (1991) Drug and alcohol abuse in patients with acute burn injuries. *Psychosomatics*, **32**, 287–293.

WELCH, C. A. (1991) Psychiatric care of the burn victim. In *Massachusetts General Hospital Handbook of General Hospital Psychiatry* (ed. N. H. Cassem) (3rd edn), pp. 465–475. St Louis: Mosby Year Book.

6 Liaison psychiatry in a large teaching hospital: the service at Leeds General Infirmary

ALLAN HOUSE

This chapter describes the work of a multidisciplinary department of liaison psychiatry based in a large teaching hospital in Leeds, a service which is unusually well developed for the UK. The aim of this paper is, therefore, to indicate the potential scope for liaison work in the NHS and to give an indication of likely workload in an established service.

Leeds health services

The Leeds metropolitan district has a population of approximately 700 000 people. Until recently it was divided into two health districts. The General Infirmary supplied services to the Leeds Western Health Authority, which served approximately 375 000 people; its ranking on the Jarman index placed it in the most socially disadvantaged third of all health districts in the country. Psychiatric in-patient services were provided to this district by the High Royds Hospital located in the village of Menston, some miles from the city centre. In Leeds Eastern Health Authority, the main hospital services were based at St James's Hospital, which unlike the General Infirmary has a large general psychiatry unit attached.

In April 1991, a major health service reorganisation was provoked by the successful applications for trust status made by the managements of both the Infirmary and St James's. The two Leeds health authorities were amalgamated into a single purchasing authority, which is now the second largest in the country. Health services are provided by the two trust hospitals and by a directly managed unit (soon to become a third wave trust). Psychiatric services for Leeds are provided by a single unit, with the exception of the department at the Infirmary which was included in the hospital's trust application.

For the purposes of this chapter, the situation prior to this reorganisation will be discussed. The figures quoted may be taken as representative of workload in a hospital dealing with a catchment area of just under 400 000, and the appropriate adjustments will need to be made to estimate likely workload in smaller health districts.

The General Infirmary at Leeds

The Infirmary is a teaching hospital with 950 beds; its associated hospitals supply a further 500 beds for medical care of the elderly, rehabilitation and a regional radiotherapy service. A number of speciality services are provided by the hospital, for example, neuro-surgery, cardiac surgery and renal medicine.

The Infirmary records approximately 25 000 hospital deaths and discharges annually. There are approximately 20 000 new out-patient attendances, 60 000 follow-up out-patient attendances and 80 000 attendances in the accident and emergency (A&E) department each year.

The only attendances which are primarily for psychiatric disorders are in the A&E department. For example, in 1989 there were 78 000 attendances in the A&E department, and 1400 (1.8%) resulted in a psychiatric diagnosis from the A&E staff. Of these, 920 were for deliberate self-harm and 480 were for other psychiatric disorders. All other psychiatric disorders seen in the hospital are identified in people who primarily attend for physical reasons, and our department makes its contacts as a result of tertiary referral from other specialists.

The liaison psychiatry department

Staffing

Liaison services to the General Infirmary and associated hospitals are provided by a multidisciplinary team, the main members of which are listed in Table 6.1. One of the consultants provides eight sessions a week of NHS time, and the other provides five sessions.

Apart from the size of the department, its most unusual feature in comparison with other UK services is the high profile of

TABLE 6.1
Staffing complement for the liaison psychiatry department
at Leeds General Infirmary (1 April 1991)

Medical
>   2 consultants – 13 sessions
>   1 tutor/registrar
>   1 senior house officer/registrar   } 1.7 WTE
>   ±1 senior registrar

Social work
>   1.5 WTE

Nursing
>   Ward based:
>   1 senior sister
>   1 junior sister
>   5 staff nurses
>   Liaison nurses:
>   1 general/A&E
>   2 behavioural nurse therapists
>   1 HIV/AIDS

Occupational therapy
>   1 senior II
>   1 basic grade

Clinical psychology
>   1 general

Secretarial/clerical
>   2 personal secretaries
>   1 part-time ward clerk

psychiatric nursing. This is partly explained by the presence of a specialist in-patient unit and partly by the active development of the role of liaison nursing.

The administrative arrangements for the department before the establishment of trust status are outlined in Fig. 6.1. Again unusually for the UK, the medical, nursing and occupational therapy budget for the department was met from the acute medical services budget and not from the mental illness unit.

The major change produced by the emergence of trust status has been in the organisation of clinical psychology services. Under the new arrangement, the General Infirmary no longer employs clinical psychology staff, although a small amount of funding is available to purchase 'contracted off' neuropsychology services. We have replaced some of the psychology function in our department by appointing a second nurse therapist with training in cognitive and behavioural therapies. Apart from the psychiatric social workers, the entire staff budget is now met by the trust.

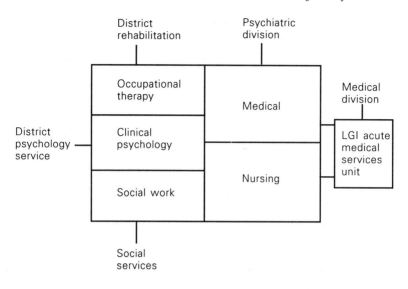

Fig. 6.1. Management arrangements before establishment of trust status (1 April 1991)

A full range of facilities is available to the department. Clinics are held in the medical out-patient department. There is a 16-bed in-patient unit in the main building of the hospital which provides for the in-patient and day-patient care of appropriate patients. Direct access to the hospital's diagnostic and treatment facilities is available to the medical staff in the department.

The referral process

Details of referrals are phoned through to the in-patient unit and entered into a ledger. The referrer is asked to give some indication of time scale for response to the referral. We undertake to see all cases referred before 10.00 a.m. during the same working day if required. More urgent cases may be referred by bleeping a medical member of the department. Non-urgent referrals or referrals for a specific person's opinion are by the personal referral slip system familiar from other areas of medical practice, or by telephone to one of the department's secretaries. In practice, the referral system stresses informality, and the majority of referrals (75–80%) are made by telephone. Out-patients are, however, referred by letter.

Direct liaison contacts are also made. The liaison nurse working in the A&E department and the nurse providing a service for patients with HIV-related disease both take direct referrals on that basis. Medical staff undertake joint liaison work with the departments of haematology, dermatology and rehabilitation.

Numbers of referrals

Recording of clinical contacts in the department has until recently not been a high priority for the hospital, and could best be described as uncoordinated. The social workers made their returns to their own social work department, the clinical psychologist to the director of the district psychology service, and the liaison nurses to the manager of the community psychiatric nursing service (despite that person not being their line manager). The medical staff collected their own information – most systematically on contacts for parasuicide assessment.

We are struggling towards a unified and more accurate system for collecting information. The parasuicide register has been computerised since 1985 and is being extended to cover all contacts; we have been successful in obtaining audit funds to develop the system further. Recent investment in a hospital-wide clinical information system makes the future look more hopeful, but we are only emerging slowly from the information Dark Ages.

Based on previous years' work, the expected number of clinical contacts for 1991 and 1992 are outlined in Table 6.2. These contacts are for psychiatry and psychology only, and do not include cases seen by the social workers or liaison nurses. Contacts on the in-patient unit (out-patient groups, drop-ins, post-discharge reviews, etc.) are not counted separately.

There are 120–150 admissions annually to the ward, which is dedicated to liaison work. After assessment, patients who require general psychiatric care are, with few exceptions, referred for admission to the appropriate general team. The majority of

TABLE 6.2
Liaison psychiatry annual referral rate at Leeds General Infirmary –
projected from 1991 figures (medical staff only)

Parasuicide assessment	750
Ward referrals (non-DSH)	250
A&E referrals (non-DSH)	250
Other contacts'	100
New out-patients	300
Total	*1650*
Follow-up out-patients	1500

admissions to the liaison ward fall into one of three groups. Firstly, there are psychiatric disorders complicating severe physical illness such as stroke or other neurological disorder, diabetes, or renal failure. (The unit provides a specialist service for HIV/AIDS cases with psychiatric disorder.) Secondly, there are psychiatric disorders complicated by physical illness. Examples include: depressive disorders where treatment is complicated by major heart disease; perforated ulcer complicating severe depression; self-inflicted stab wounds resulting from paranoid illness. Both these groups may be initially bedbound and require levels of physical care which cannot be provided on most acute psychiatric admissions wards, such as intravenous fluids, medication for physical disorders or daily physiotherapy. The third major group of admissions consists of patients with severe and usually chronic somatisation, who are admitted most frequently to treat immobility, loss of functions, drug overuse or associated mood disorder. Such patients require special nursing skills, individually-tailored programmes and a therapeutic milieu which cannot be provided on acute psychiatric admissions wards.

The purpose of this chapter is not to describe the nature of liaison practice and we will not therefore go into more details of types of clinical problem seen. Suffice it to say the pattern of our referrals is very similar to that described from other UK services. In other words, the majority of our referrals come from the general medical service, deliberate self-harm assessment and the A&E department. In contrast, general and special surgical teams refer relatively few cases. Where liaison links have been established (haematology, dermatology, rehabilitation) referral rates are higher. For local reasons, referral rates from obstetrics and gynaecology and oncology (other than haematology) are remarkably low. Between 3 and 4% of referrals for deliberate self-harm live outside Leeds, as do 6–8% of other referrals.

The main dilemma: deciding on the style of service

The principal aim of our service is to provide a system for assessment and management of psychiatric disorder which is rapid and efficient in its response and comprehensive in its availability to the hospital. The referral system is informal and there is telephone and bleep access to a doctor and a liaison nurse at all times. The resulting referrals include many acute problems from the medical wards and A&E department.

This emphasis on rapid and comprehensive service provision does not sit easily within our working style, which is based on close liaison with individual departments, specialisation and long-term involvement with severe and intractable problems. The typical referral would be the chronic somatising patient or somebody with persistent difficulties adjusting to chronic physical illness.

Providing both types of service is one of the major headaches to be faced in running a liaison service. It is tempting to dispense with one, and some argue that the acute work is not a proper function of a liaison service. It is frequently unpopular, especially when parasuicide assessment is undertaken in a poorly organised or unsupervised manner. It is difficult to operate on a sessional basis, and it appears unspecialised. However, the efficient organisation of the acute work is much appreciated by the general hospital staff and it is these short-order and unpredictable referrals which general psychiatrists find most difficult to fit into their routine. On the other hand, the more chronic and difficult cases – somatising and poor adjustment to physical illness particularly – require more specialist skill in their management, and although fewer in number they can be expensive (in time and money) and exasperating to the non-psychiatrists who treat them.

Liaison psychiatry has to look in two directions when justifying its existence, and it is unlikely to have many friends if it neither meets the needs of the general hospital nor reduces the workload of the rest of the psychiatric service. These conflicting demands must be resolved in the planning and provision of a liaison service, even when it is to be provided on a part-time or sessional basis.

7 Providing a psychiatric service to a large cancer hospital

PETER MAGUIRE and
PENELOPE HOPWOOD

This chapter presents the reasons why patients with cancer require specialised psychiatric services. It describes the ways in which research has identified effective management and led to the development of services to meet these needs. Finally, it describes the psychiatric service provided in a regional cancer hospital.

Why target patients with cancer?

Up to 30% of patients who have cancer develop a moderately severe or severe affective disorder as a result of diagnosis or treatment (Greer, 1985). A similar proportion develop body-image problems and sexual difficulties (Maguire, 1985). Body-image problems include a loss of physical integrity, heightened self-consciousness, and a feeling of being less feminine or masculine.

The use of radiotherapy and chemotherapy increases the risk of psychiatric morbidity through adverse side-effects like fatigue, nausea and vomiting. Up to 25% of patients on chemotherapy develop conditioned responses. Thus any stimulus, sight, sound or smell which reminds them of treatment causes them to experience reflexively nausea and/or vomiting. Such conditioning can lead to phobic reactions and failure to complete treatment. Confusional states are also relatively common because of cancer progression and spread, metabolic changes and effects of treatment (Maguire, 1985). Without intervention, much of this psychiatric morbidity persists over time since the factors that provoked onset, like fear of recurrence or failure to adapt to an altered body image, are still present (Maguire *et al*, 1980).

Surely they are helped already?

Data about high rates of psychological and psychiatric morbidity in patients with cancer have been available for over a decade. Surely, therefore, clinicians involved in cancer care already recognise and treat these patients or make appropriate psychiatric referrals? Unfortunately this is not so, and both parties contribute to low recognition and referral rates.

Patients with cancer believe, albeit wrongly, that these problems are an inevitable consequence of their predicament. Since they also believe that they cannot be resolved, there is no point in mentioning them to a doctor or nurse. Moreover, they do not want to burden staff whom they like and respect. They appreciate that the staff are hard-pressed already and might view disclosure of problems as due to ingratitude or inadequacy. They perceive doctors and nurses to be primarily concerned with physical aspects of care, and that it is not legitimate to disclose other concerns.

For their part, doctors and nurses rarely ask the kinds of question that promote disclosure (e.g. "how have you felt about losing a breast?", "how do you see your treatment working out?"). Instead, they use distancing tactics like *normalisation* ("you are bound to be upset"), *premature reassurance* ("don't worry, we will get you well in no time") or *switching* where they change the topic immediately. They do this because of genuine fears that psychological enquiry will unleash strong emotions which will harm patients and be difficult to contain. It could also encourage patients to ask difficult questions like "is it cancer?" or "am I ever going to recover?" and bring the health professional too close to the patient's true predicament.

These barriers to communication have a serious effect. At best, only 20% of patients who develop psychological and psychiatric morbidity are recognised as needing help (Maguire *et al*, 1980). Even when a psychiatric liaison service was provided to a medical oncology ward, only 40% of those needing help because of a depressive illness were recognised, helped or psychiatrically referred (Hardman *et al*, 1989).

Overcoming these barriers

A traditional liaison psychiatry service relying on doctor-led referrals will see few of those patients and relatives who most need help. Instead, they may see 'distressed' patients who do not merit intervention. We adopted, therefore, two additional strategies: the use of specialist nurses in the short term, and longer term training in assessment skills of doctors and nurses involved in cancer care.

Use of specialist nurses

On an experimental basis, we employed and trained a specialist nurse to counsel and monitor women undergoing mastectomy for breast cancer. She had a strong nursing background in cancer care rather than psychiatry, as she needed to be credible to her patients.

After a three month training period using demonstration video-tapes, practising assessment and counselling with real patients and being given feedback, she was able to recognise and refer 90% or more of those patients who needed psychiatric help. Subsequently, she recognised and referred 75% of those patients who developed psychological or psychiatric morbidity and were randomly allocated to her care (Maguire *et al*, 1980). In contrast, only 15% of patients in the control group were recognised and referred.

Importantly, the effectiveness of the subsequent intervention led to a four-fold reduction in psychological and psychiatric morbidity in the specialist nurse's group (Maguire *et al*, 1980). However, the monitoring of this target group was time-consuming since patients were assessed at home every two months after discharge. The nurse was also faced with a steadily accumulating patient load. Some women were made more anxious by a visit because it reactivated their worries about cancer.

Alternative systems

In a further randomised controlled trial (Wilkinson *et al*, 1988) our original monitoring system was compared with two alternatives:

(a) *A limited intervention scheme* where the specialist nurse made only one monitoring home visit within six weeks of discharge from hospital after surgery for breast cancer. Patients found to have psychiatric problems were referred appropriately. Those without problems were asked to get in touch if problems arose later.

(b) *A ward nurse/community scheme* which relied on ward nurses to monitor patients' adjustment and refer the patient after discharge to the appropriate community nurse. Both ward and community nurses were first trained in the relevant assessment skills (Faulkner & Maguire, 1984).

While the ward/community scheme had little impact, the psychological and psychiatric morbidity was as much reduced in the limited intervention group as in the full intervention group (Wilkinson *et al*, 1988). This model has now been adopted for use with other specialist nurses, including those involved with patients with lymphoma, cervical cancer, and heterogeneous groups of patients.

This more economic use of specialist nurses' time has enabled them to take on more therapeutic roles like teaching patients anxiety management techniques or using cognitive therapy. However, it carries certain risks, especially the possibility that other health professionals will be tempted to leave all psychological care to specialist nurses. The longer term strategy has been to train doctors and nurses involved in cancer care in psychological assessment skills.

Developing the service

The research findings concerning psychiatric morbidity, problems in detection and the role of specialist nurses prompted the Cancer Research Campaign (CRC) to establish a psychological medicine group at the Christie Hospital. The Christie is a 350-bed cancer hospital which serves the North West Region. The group is accommodated in a refurbished house opposite the main out-patient department.

The main objectives of the CRC group are to develop and evaluate ways of improving the psychological and psychiatric care of cancer patients and their relatives. Its establishment has enabled us to provide a liaison psychiatry service as well as to conduct relevant research.

The CRC initially funded one consultant post (PH) and a research registrar post, while the University of Manchester funded the group's director (PM) and a second consultant. The CRC took over the funding of this second consultant post in November 1991. The Christie now funds a full-time clinical secretary and provides the accommodation. An average of 11 new patient referrals per week come from medical staff at the Christie, other consultants within the Greater Manchester area, general practitioners locally and beyond, and specialist cancer nurses both within and outside the South Manchester Health Authority.

The liaison service (supervised by PH) accepts medical referrals of in-patients, day patients and out-patients at the Christie. It also receives referrals from two research nurses who are employed to assess quality of life in clinical trials. The group director (PM) also receives medical referrals from Christie but concentrates on the growing number of referrals from specialist cancer nurses and general practitioners. The specialist nurses are encouraged to develop further their assessment, counselling and therapeutic skills through supervision and attending university courses.

Evaluation

The staff split their time equally between clinical and research work. A study of consecutively referred patients has shown that 80% of them recover completely. We are now undertaking research to see if we can prevent psychiatric disorder through early identification of and intervention in those at risk. Potentially useful indicators include the number of unresolved concerns, low self-esteem and adverse effects of treatment. We are continuing to evaluate ways of helping medical and nursing staff improve their ability to recognise patients who need psychological help.

Our willingness to provide a prompt clinical service has fostered cooperation with our research. Feedback of our research findings has, in turn, enhanced clinical care.

References

FAULKNER, A. & MAGUIRE, P. (1984) Teaching ward nurses to monitor cancer patients. *Clinical Oncology*, **10**, 583–589.

GREER, S. (1985) Cancer: psychiatric aspects. In *Recent Advances in Clinical Psychiatry* (ed. K. Granville Grossman), pp. 87–104. London: Churchill Livingstone.

HARDMAN, A., MAGUIRE, P. & CROWTHER, D. (1989) The recognition of psychiatric morbidity on a medical oncology ward. *Journal of Psychosomatic Research*, **33**, 235–239.

MAGUIRE, P. (1985) Psychological impact of cancer. *British Journal of Hospital Medicine*, **34**, 100–103.

——, TAIT, A., BROOKE, M., *et al* (1980) The effect of counselling on the psychiatric morbidity associated with mastectomy. *British Medical Journal*, **281**, 1454–1456.

WILKINSON, S., MAGUIRE, P. & TAIT, A. (1988) Life after breast cancer. *Nursing Times*, **84**, 34–37.

8 A child psychiatry liaison service

PETER LOADER

A dictionary definition of 'liaison' includes 'association, cooperation', 'an illicit sexual relationship' and 'coordination and cooperation between two units or allied armies, or between higher and lower commands'. A liaison officer is 'an officer acting to link between units, armies and commands'. Liaison appears to involve a particular type of association where cooperation cannot be taken for granted, is problematic or viewed as suspect or even inappropriate. In medicine, I see liaison work as joining different domains or concepts of human function (e.g. mind and body; psychology and biology), rather than prioritising either one. There seems to be something inherently worrying about such work, such that it is often understated or even secret. A liaison of views on human problems is not easy, since allegiance to one particular perspective is the rule, and is often encouraged. Holding one view or another may be an advantage in attempting to understand the complexities of human functioning, which may otherwise seem overwhelming, so that we may achieve some feeling of mastery.

The tendency to divide human functioning into different levels results in different scientific disciplines. These include: sociology and anthropology (focusing on society); family therapy (focusing on the family); communication theory (focusing on one-to-one relationships); psychology (focusing on the individual); and biology (focusing on the body). There is overlap between these, but it takes a lot of effort to become competent in any of them and we tend to train in one and then spend our working lives there. Each level of study and practice has its own clubs, journals and conferences; people in each rarely talk to each other, an activity which is not helped by the development of different professional languages. While this stratification has allowed great advances in particular fields, there is a risk that we forget that in real life these different levels do not exist; rather, there is a complex but coherent whole. The fact is that we are all interested in the same thing – human functioning and human problems – and are merely looking from different vantage points.

The clinical service

I spend three liaison sessions each week in a general hospital, the Whittington Hospital in Islington, London[1]. There I am part of the Child and Family Psychiatric Service, a small team made up of two consultant child psychiatrists (each with three sessions), a senior registrar in child psychiatry (four sessions) and two seconded social workers (one full-time, one part-time). In the past we accepted referrals from within or without the hospital but now only from within. Most of our referrals come from paediatricians but some come from other departments, such as adult psychiatry.

Consultation or liaison?

Much of my time in liaison work has little to do with liaison as defined above, but is spent seeing patients passed on by other doctors because the problem has been deemed to be primarily psychiatric. This work is important but, in my experience, often involves very little association between the different approaches of medicine and psychiatry, or between the different professionals involved. Such association is difficult, not only because of the different interests and languages but because it also seems expensive and time consuming, although in reality this may not be so. It is here, in the interplay between these different points of view, and different kinds of doctor, that the creativity and excitement of liaison work lies.

However, the time taken up by seeing patients referred to our team involves some liaison work. This may range from an exchange of letters, through corridor discussions, to a feedback discussion at our liaison meeting. I see these patients either on my own or with another member of the team. Very occasionally I see them together with the referrer, usually a paediatrician, but this is unusual and makes me feel particularly anxious. I worry that I am taking up valuable paediatric time, although this has never been apparent

---

1.The author is no longer based at the Whittington Hospital (see contributor list).

from their comments. Perhaps, in this personal inhibition, lies a common liaison problem that arises when two people have different approaches to problems – or think that they do. There is a fear that one's own approach may be misunderstood, not valued, or perhaps is inappropriate to the referrer's needs. I think this is a common problem in liaison work, although perhaps less so in child psychiatry than in its adult counterpart. Working with children promotes liaison and I think this reflects the way that children demand to be seen – beautifully reflected in the paediatrician Apley's comment that "the sick child is ill all over". Children promote an 'all over', integrated approach to illness and health.

The liaison meeting

The weekly liaison meeting, previously called the psychosocial meeting, is for me the lynch-pin of my liaison work. It takes place in the paediatric department, lasts for one-and-a-half hours and is attended by the whole child psychiatry liaison team, paediatricians, nurses, representatives of the physiotherapists, speech therapists, dieticians, health visitors and teachers from the hospital school. It is a large group and an expensive meeting. It used to consider all the children on the paediatric ward and was firmly run by the chief paediatrician, who wanted to check that the children and their families were 'plugged-in' to the appropriate services. His retirement and the arrival of two new consultants led to a change in the form of the meeting. Now ward and out-patients are selected for discussion, mostly by the paediatricians but also by other professional groups.

The meeting is very lively and may appear rather disorganised. The discussion has to be framed in language that everyone can understand. Although there is a rough agenda, we rarely get through all of it and may spend all the time talking about one child or a particular quandary that somebody has experienced. There is a confluence of many different sources of information, perspectives and points of view, which sometimes ends in disagreement. At other times it is extremely creative, producing new understandings of problems or innovative plans of action.

There is a pecking order of sorts, but given the hierarchy-bound hospital system, we have developed a forum where everybody feels able to contribute. The most helpful contributions often come from the most unlikely sources. The meeting is given a very high priority by the paediatricians, and this is important for its success.

It is the spirit of this meeting that I want to emphasise, for this is the essence of liaison work. It brings together professionals with different experiences and points of view and allows us to have a conversation that confronts the complexity of our patients' problems, and ultimately enhances the quality of their care.

The joint clinic

Another aspect of my liaison work is an asthma clinic, run jointly with a consultant paediatrician. This started as an experimental venture and reflected our mutual interest in the psychological aspects of childhood asthma. My colleagues agreed to take on more than their share of the referrals while I spent an entire weekly session (a third of my time at the hospital) in this liaison task.

Initially I sat in on the clinic (feeling rather like a medical student), watching the paediatrician and occasionally making a psychologically orientated comment. Gradually I became more confident and more involved as I realised that the paediatrician was spending a lot of time in my kind of territory. The patients appeared to like this arrangement. Previously the paediatrician had noticed a marked resistance to psychiatric referral but now parents began to complain about not seeing the psychiatrist when I was unable to be there. Another interesting feature was that parents would say quite different things to each of us. They would freely tell me about problems in their family life which would be side-stepped when asked about (and skilfully so) by the paediatrician. They might even direct answers to questions from him to me. As time went by, he became more psychologically orientated while I became more and more aware of the physical aspects. At times I would even warn him not to overemphasise psychological and family considerations.

Time was a problem. The clinic grew longer and longer and eventually we decided that I should sit in the next room and see selected patients for whom psychological factors appeared to be of particular importance. This worked reasonably well but the liaison factor was obviously markedly reduced. We tried to meet to discuss these patients but there never seemed to be enough time. This illustrates a very real problem with liaison work. We enjoyed working together and the patients benefited, but it was time consuming. Even with the cooperation and support of colleagues, our joint clinic did not achieve the expected throughput of patients.

Joint training

Joint training is another aspect of the liaison work of the Child and Family Psychiatric Service. We have presented examples of our work at hospital and paediatric meetings. We have also presented, with the paediatricians, patients with whom we have worked either separately or together.

Joint training in interview skills embodies the aspects of liaison work which I am emphasising here. This started as an initiative of the primary care department, which arranged a day for hospital consultants to address this neglected aspect of training. Mock interviews involved actors and staff role-playing patients, and afterwards videotapes were played back for detailed discussion. Later, a half-day course was arranged for the paediatric firm, including medical students, together with the child psychiatrists. In small groups, we role-played a number of scenarios, such as breaking bad news. The videotape was played back and discussed, with the 'doctor' saying what he was trying to do, the 'patient' saying what the interview was like for him/her and observers adding their views.

We learnt a great deal from each other, particularly about how complex even a short interview can be. This training revealed just how important it is for a doctor to have interpersonal skills as well as diagnostic ones. Getting information depends not only on asking the right questions but on asking them in the right way. The exercise requires a lot of trust between colleagues and results in a healthy respect for each other's skills. It also provides a powerful method of teaching the most basic skill for all doctors – the clinical interview. Further training is planned as a regular event, involving the child psychiatrists and other departments. Although this is a very small part of my work, I include it here because it fosters an increased understanding of different clinical tasks and encourages a broader view of illness. A real development of liaison work will require enhanced opportunities for training, and must involve practical experiences such as this.

Ward liaison

Another potentially time-consuming aspect of liaison psychiatry is work with in-patients. Within the three sessions available, it has not previously been possible for me to provide this sort of service. However, I and one of the social workers from our team have now planned to commit ourselves to a regular hour-a-week slot on the children's ward. We need to have a ward presence, to get a feel of the ward and to be seen to be available there. We will be available to talk to the nurses and other staff, and to children and their parents.

Conclusions

In this brief chapter, I have tried to emphasise my approach to the *liaison* task. This involves more than the provision of a consultation service by seeing referred patients, although, in practice, this usually constitutes the bulk of the work. A liaison service must also promote an interchange of points of view, or a *conversation* between professionals who see human problems from different vantage points. As my child psychiatrist colleague on the liaison team puts it, we must be 'a department without walls'.

In my experience it is this aspect of liaison work that is most understated, both in clinical services and in training. Perhaps this is not surprising given the time constraints of all professional groups working in the hospital setting, but it probably also reflects the difficulty of the task. Different disciplines focus on different aspects of human functioning and have different jobs to do, so that a conversation between them is no easy affair. In addition, there is an increasing pressure to justify our work by seeing enough cases, with little appreciation of time spent talking to each other. As with the popular sense of the term 'affair', the development of this aspect of liaison work may depend not only on whether we want to get together in this way, but also whether we are allowed to.

9 Liaison services for elderly people

SUSAN MARY BENBOW

People over the age of 65 occupy half of all NHS hospital beds at any one time and therefore their management represents a major cost to the health service. Their treatment is complicated by the fact that both their physical and mental disorders tend to have different characteristics compared with the same illnesses suffered by younger people.

A further problem is that mental and physical illnesses are particularly liable to occur together in late life. Elderly people with depressive disorders often have associated physical illness (Dover & McWilliam, 1992) and increased mortality (Murphy *et al*, 1988), so the treatment of physical disorders is likely to demand considerable attention and time in the old age psychiatry department. Conversely, a number of reports testify to the increased risk of mental disorders in the elderly who are physically ill, with either acute (O'Riordan *et al*, 1989; Ramsay *et al*, 1991) or chronic disorders (Sadavoy *et al*, 1990; Shah *et al*, 1992). Many people over the age of 65 on general medical and surgical wards have mental disorders; dementia has been found in up to 30% and delirium in up to 25% (Pitt, 1993). Depression has been reported to be the best predictor of somatic discomfort in the elderly (Rozzini *et al*, 1988). In these circumstances, even physicians who have some experience of the management of mental disorders in the elderly are likely to require the close cooperation and support of their psychiatrist colleagues.

What then is the extent of need for psychiatric services for patients in other departments of the general hospital? How can systems be established to ensure that elderly people receive an effective liaison service?

Developing a new service in Central Manchester

The start of the service

Over the first year after I was appointed as an old age psychiatrist, 35% of my 322 referrals came from doctors working in general hospitals. I did not actively seek to promote liaison referrals but I had established links with the geriatric physicians, personally and through a weekly joint out-patient clinic. Referrals were seen mainly on a consultation basis on their wards or in the community after discharge. Medical colleagues provided similar consultations in return. Of all liaison consultations requested by the hospital, 58% were from geriatric physicians. The two main diagnostic groups were dementias (32% of liaison referrals) and affective illnesses (27%) (Benbow, 1987).

This system relied on referral by the physician or surgeon and (in most cases) agreement on behalf of the patient to see the psychiatrist. At that time, out-of-area referrals accounted for 21% of liaison referrals. The policy regarding GP referrals was not to accept referrals from outside Central Manchester, because it was difficult to ensure continuity of psychiatric care.

A review of liaison referrals over that first year impressed upon me that this work constituted a large part of an old age psychiatrist's workload, even without seeking unrecognised psychiatric illnesses.

Increasing referral rates

Since the first year, the percentage of referrals from hospital doctors to the old age psychiatry service in Central Manchester has increased further, to 52% of the 392 referrals in 1989–90. From 1985, two consultants shared the provision of this service. The changes are summarised in Table 9.1, which relates the numbers of referrals to the catchment area population aged 65 years and above (17 400). During this five year period, there has been a 23% increase in total referrals, and this is accounted for entirely by the increase in liaison referrals, while the number of referrals from the community has hardly changed. The liaison referral rate per thousand of the elderly population has almost doubled.

Interpretation of the data is not straightforward. The referral rates do not take into account cross-boundary flows. Not all of the liaison referrals seen in Central Manchester are for people resident in the catchment area. In addition, some elderly residents will have their physical disorders treated at hospitals outside our catchment area and will be referred to other liaison services.

TABLE 9.1
Referral patterns to the old age psychiatry service in Central Manchester, 1985–90

Year	Total number of referrals	Liaison referrals	% liaison referrals	Liaison referral rate/1000
1985–86	380	135	36	7.8
1986–87	369	164	44	9.4
1987–88	439	203	46	11.7
1988–89	386	191	49	11.0
1989–90	469	241	51	13.9

Although these figures provide an indication of conspicuous morbidity, they cannot be considered in isolation from factors which influence referral, such as availability of services and the sensitivity of geriatric physicians to psychiatric problems. One recent study found that geriatricians were aware of only 42% of those who were depressed (Pitt, 1993). Dementia is commonly not identified in patients on general medical wards (Folks & Ford, 1985; Feldman *et al*, 1987). Although screening for dementia and depression might improve case identification (Pitt, 1993), it is questionable whether available services could respond to these unmet needs.

In absolute terms, the number of liaison referrals per year has increased from 135 to 241 over the five year period. New referrals (those never seen previously) ranged from 100 to 180. Thus in an average week there would be a minimum of two new liaison referrals plus one other patient already known to the service who required reassessment. At times there have been up to nine referrals weekly. Sessions are not set aside for this work because that would sometimes result in delays before patients were seen. In addition there is the fear of being swamped by a potential increase in referrals that might arise from the many beds available to the geriatricians. At least one session per week, and sometimes up to three sessions, of consultant old age psychiatrists' time has been spent seeing in-patients referred from other hospital doctors. This does not take into account the additional time devoted to following these patients up after the initial assessment, usually by seeing them in their homes after discharge from hospital. Seeing patients in the joint geriatric/psychogeriatric out-patient clinic, with one of the geriatric physicians, accounts for another session each week. Thus a minimum of three sessions a week (and sometimes far more) of the consultant old age psychiatrists' time is spent providing this liaison service, which does not include some of the other aspects of liaison psychiatry that are described below.

Limited resources

Other staff contribute to the care of these patients, who may receive further assessment and treatment in the day-hospital, as in-patients in the old-age psychiatry unit, or in the community. This may involve secretarial and administrative staff, nurses, occupational and speech therapists, physiotherapists and clinical psychologists, in any of these settings. These staff are part of the old age psychiatry service, but they do not have time allocated specifically for the liaison service.

Although half our referrals originate from the liaison service, our orientation is still towards community work, and I suspect that this tends to pressurise the time available to see people referred for liaison consultations. Assigning sessions for liaison psychiatry might be one way of recognising and providing a better service for this aspect of our work.

Apart from medical time, the main resource limitations that I have been aware of relate to the medical and surgical wards, which have had very little access to occupational therapy unless it is provided by staff in the old age psychiatry unit, and this is not always appropriate. Similarly, social work input on the medical and surgical wards has been limited, but it should not be necessary to refer patients to a psychiatrist so that they can see a social worker. Better provision of these resources to our colleagues would make it possible for the liaison old age psychiatrist to work more effectively.

Generally, only about 10-15% of people referred for liaison consultation in our district are admitted to a psychiatric bed. Of these, some will have presented with deliberate self-harm. The others are usually people with very complex medical and psychiatric problems, and the death rate among this group is high.

Ideally, psychiatric department staff should be present when case conferences are held on medical or surgical wards, and vice versa, in order that all those involved contribute to management plans. Staffing limitations usually make this impractical, within our available resources. An alternative would be to appoint a liaison nurse with responsibility for linking medical and psychiatric teams and ensuring that joint management plans are carried out in the community, following discharge.

Working with geriatricians

The joint out-patient clinic has continued since my appointment to the service, although its function has evolved throughout, partly due to changes in the geriatricians who have been involved. Usually the two consultants see the patient and any relative together.

It can be a sobering experience to witness the patient directing psychiatric symptoms to the psychiatrist and physical ones to the physician. My experience suggests that how the two consultants work together is critical. Some geriatricians have been more enthusiastic than others, perhaps with an interest in particular problems. Some have regularly admitted patients to medical wards from the clinic. Others have preferred to negotiate provision of medical problem management for people admitted to the psychiatric wards. I have seen both models work. Some geriatric physicians have preferred to follow up patients in their own medical clinics after joint assessment and discussion. Others have seen people in the joint clinic for follow-up appointments. Responsibility for both immediate and longer term care may need to be negotiated, and some geriatricians will feel happier than others in dealing with patients they perceive as primarily suffering from psychiatric illness. Some geriatricians are better psychiatrists than others – and I assume that the same is true of the medical skills of psychiatrists.

We used to have regular meetings of consultants in geriatric medicine and old age psychiatry to discuss matters of mutual interest, but these seemed to become less important when a joint care planning group for the elderly was established, providing a forum for these issues. Our multi-disciplinary lunchtime teaching session attracts staff from geriatric medicine, particularly from their day hospital.

Education and training

Attempts have been made to arrange joint meetings for continuing medical education. Joint medical and clinical audit, and research involving each others' patients, present further opportunities for collaboration. Such activities would be facilitated by allocating sessions to liaison work.

Teaching is another aspect of the old age psychiatry liaison service which needs to be recognised. During their psychiatric clerkship, undergraduate medical students have accompanied me on consultations. Sometimes they interview the patients first, then discuss them with me and join me at my subsequent interview with the patients. Most students have been enthusiastic about this teaching and indicated that they had learnt a lot. Many of the patients seen on the geriatric wards are ideally suited to teaching undergraduates about the complex interactions of physical and mental disorders. This teaching might be particularly effective if provided jointly by psychiatrists and geriatricians, but there has not often been time to do this.

Post-graduates on the psychiatric training rotation see liaison referrals, with supervision, and this is an essential part of their old age psychiatry training. Higher trainees may also attend the joint clinic, if a patient with whom they are involved is attending, so that the clinic also contributes to their training. Higher training for old age psychiatry also provides other opportunities relevant to liaison psychiatry, including sessions working with geriatricians and in neuropsychiatry.

Benefits of liaison services

One of the main arguments in favour of developing a liaison service relies on the considerable overlap between physical and psychiatric illnesses in the elderly: here we have a population of elderly people whom we know have a higher psychiatric morbidity than the general population. Therefore liaison psychiatrists have to develop special skills in the assessment and treatment of physically ill people.

There is evidence that unrecognised psychiatric illness in elderly in-patients is likely to lengthen hospital stay (Lipowski, 1983) and that identification and treatment of mental disorders can reduce it. Disturbed behaviour may interfere with management of physical illness and delay recovery (Millar, 1981). Length of stay may reduce if a liaison psychiatrist is involved (Levitan & Kornfeld, 1981) and it has been argued that these advantages ensure that a liaison service will be cost-effective. A study of elderly patients with hip fractures on surgical wards evaluated the effect of routine psychiatric screening shortly after admission, followed by psychiatric consultation where appropriate (Strain *et al*, 1991). About 60% of these patients were found to have a psychiatric diagnosis. Following psychiatric intervention, the mean length of stay was reduced by two days and the reduction in hospital costs greatly exceeded the cost of the psychiatric service that was provided.

Thus a service which facilitates treatment of physical and psychiatric problems simultaneously may shorten the length of stay, reduce costs and improve the quality of care. It may ensure that psychiatric expertise is provided at a relatively early stage to those who otherwise would not receive its benefit. It may prevent recurrence and long-term morbidity. It may also prevent mis-placement, particularly unnecessary nursing home placements (Lichtenstein & Winograd, 1984).

Liaison work with the elderly can also present serious challenges for old age psychiatrists. Often only limited information is available on patients seen in medical wards. Information based on assessment of the home environment and from family or neighbours, which would be routinely gathered in the course of community-based work, is not easily available and this requires considerable extra time. While there are some useful ward-based observations, they provide little guidance on how patients have been functioning in their own homes. Sometimes physicians assume that disability seen in the unfamiliar environment of the ward will inevitably persist elsewhere, and may be reluctant to discharge patients to their own homes. Other problems arising from inappropriate attitudes and practices in the management of the elderly on general wards have been reviewed recently (Pitt, 1993).

Purchasers may be impressed with the argument that a liaison service improves quality of life and decreases length of stay. Doctors in other specialities may be more interested in the argument of improvement in their outcome indicators and prevention of misplacement. Colleagues in the department of psychiatry may be pleased by the improvement in training and teaching if liaison services are developed, and the non-specific benefits of closer relationships with colleagues in medicine and surgery. Many old age psychiatrists have found that they can rely on the support of geriatric medical colleagues when in competition with other departments over resources.

The underlying principles

Old age psychiatrists have a major advantage in providing liaison services on medical and surgical wards: elderly people are present throughout the general hospital, but the majority of them are on geriatric wards and most requests for liaison psychiatry services come from their geriatric medical colleagues. Thus the service needs to take account of a high demand from one area (geriatric medicine) and a more diffuse demand from other departments.

The British Geriatrics Society and the Section of Old Age Psychiatry of the Royal College of Psychiatrists (Murdoch & Montgomery, 1992) recently agreed an updated set of guidelines for liaison between geriatric physicians and psychiatrists. All old age psychiatry consultants and managers should consider the extent to which these guidelines have already been implemented, and plan to remedy any deficits. The guidelines should also prove valuable to those who purchase services and those who audit them. They set out the principles of a good service, but this does not imply that there is only one 'right way' to implement them. Flexibility is often a key requirement.

The guidelines set out 16 important principles which can assist planning and implementation of services. These are summarised and discussed below:

1. **"Specialist health services for the elderly should be a unity for 'consumers' ... Transfers should be smooth and mutually agreed ... to ensure the most appropriate management for patients."**

For the consumers of services it is important that a 'seamless' service is provided. Elderly people may present inappropriately, for example by being referred to a physician with what is essentially a psychiatric condition. Services should be planned to ensure that they are directed easily and quickly to a more appropriate service. This implies that referral systems need to exist to ensure provision of appropriate treatment in medical, surgical and psychiatric settings. Various different models exist to this end. Some districts may have a joint out-patient clinic where people can be seen by both a psychiatrist and a geriatric physician. This allows both specialists to sort out which service might most appropriately manage someone with physical and psychological problems. Alternatively they might agree to continue joint management in the clinic for some people with mixed or complex problems. A joint clinic helps to provide a unified service to out-patients but does not facilitate liaison for in-patients. However, if the two specialists meet regularly, they will have a forum for discussing mutual problems and this may encourage cross-consultations or joint assessments outside the clinic.

Some districts run joint assessment wards where both physician and psychiatrist have admission rights and staff are from both backgrounds (Pitt & Silver, 1982). This prevents repeated transfer between services (Brown & McEvoy,1993). Sometimes one specialist might regularly attend the ward round or case conferences of the other; a senior registrar in geriatric medicine attended ward rounds on the psychogeriatric assessment ward where I trained. Each model has different implications in terms of service development. Attending ward rounds of the sibling speciality is time-consuming, and where geriatric physicians have many patients it is impossible to be other than selective, in which case a seamless service might be provided for patients on one ward but not those on another.

2. **"Unity does not mean blurring of the specificity of the particular professions and facilities within the service or the patients' right of access to them."**

Thus physicians will still care primarily for medically ill people and psychiatrists for the mentally ill. If a mentally ill old person can be assessed and a treatment plan made while inadvertently admitted to a medical bed, this should not mean that they should remain there for treatment. Mechanisms between the specialities should ensure that people are treated in the appropriate treatment setting, although there will be occasions when it is debatable whether this will be psychiatric or medical. For most people, the geriatrician and psychiatrist will agree together which setting is most appropriate and two further guidelines state how this should be determined:

3. **"Responsibility should be determined by the assessed clinical and care needs of the patient ..."**
4. **"The currently assessed clinical needs of patients at home rather than their past medical or psychiatric history should determine their referral and placement."**

Current assessment will take into account physical and psychiatric problems. My own view is that sometimes, although the reason for admission is clearly medical and, of itself, merits admission to a medical or surgical ward, there may be concurrent psychiatric problems and the person might be better managed on a psychiatric ward, even though the psychiatric problems alone would not have necessitated admission.

> **Case example**
> Miss B was in her late eighties, suffered from Alzheimer's disease, and had been known for a number of years to both the old age psychiatry service and the geriatricians. She was an independent woman who refused services and was considered to be demanding and uncooperative. She developed a series of medical problems, (including heart failure, chest infections and falls) and was admitted to medical wards as an emergency on several occasions. Each time, the medical staff were anxious about her discharge home and she was referred for a consultation. We agreed to deal with her future medical problems; this gave us the opportunity to introduce her to the day hospital while an in-patient. We hoped that this might allow closer monitoring of her physical health, perhaps preventing further medical or psychiatric admissions. This management plan was successful for many months.

I would argue for comprehensive assessment by physician and psychiatrist of the person's current difficulties and needs, and flexibility in the subsequent arrangements for care.

5. "Patients [who] fall into a 'grey area' ... become a matter for negotiation between the two services ... No patient should be allowed to 'fall between two stools'."

Some people have mixed problems and it is not easy to determine where treatment should take place. If there are close links between them, the two specialists may see the person together, either in hospital, or by carrying out a joint home visit, and can then negotiate an agreed plan. If it becomes clear that the alternative setting might have been more appropriate then rapid reconsideration should occur, since another basic premise should be that:

6. "Speedy systems of cross-referral ... should be established."

To rely on written referral between specialities is inappropriate, although it might be adequate for non-urgent out-patient referrals. Most referrals should be made by telephone, and are facilitated by familiarity with the other person involved. Where an urgent response relies on a 'duty doctor' system, it should be possible for the duty doctor to avail themselves of specialist advice. It is accepted in old age psychiatry that people will be seen by a consultant on an urgent domiciliary visit in the community, but in many hospitals, if a person on a medical or surgical ward needs urgent psychiatric assessment, it will be one of the most junior psychiatrists who answers the call. This is another way in which patients referred from other wards may receive a second class service, and is another area which will need consideration in planning services. The dilemma is how to ensure a rapid response by a specialist of appropriate seniority both for people in the community and those in hospital. Many districts may have no old age psychiatrist or only one, who is struggling to provide a community service to a disproportionately large population.

7. "Assessment by physicians in geriatric medicine and psychiatrists in the care of the elderly must be included as an essential component of services ... Liaison ... should be included in 'job plans', 'service agreements' and 'business plans'."

Thus, old age psychiatrists should negotiate reciprocal liaison systems with their geriatric colleagues and have sessional time allocated for carrying out this work. If time is not allocated, elderly mentally ill people on medical wards will often have to be seen on a consultation basis, and they may receive a second class service. This is a particular problem now that it is customary for old age psychiatrists to spend the bulk of their time in the community. There is a danger that community referrals will be given higher priority as their needs are unknown. One could argue the reverse: that people on geriatric medical wards are already receiving care, and, if inappropriately placed, they may be using unnecessary and costly health service resources. A financial argument can be made therefore for giving in-patients higher priority for assessment and treatment. Realistically, a service will need to be planned which takes account of the needs of both groups.

It is essential to allocate at least one consultant session per week to work with medical and surgical in-patients, in addition to work with the department of geriatric medicine. In a district with a large population and many general hospital beds, there will be several old age psychiatrists and it might be desirable to negotiate for one of them to take special responsibility for the overall organisation of the liaison service. This would focus the majority of liaison sessions on one post and would ensure that this aspect of the service received appropriate recognition.

8.   "Adequate resources ... are required ... Inadequate resources inhibit collaboration."

This is self-evident, but is the reality of service provision for most people. If staffing is inadequate, how are priorities to be set? If we try to provide a service to everyone, the risk is that no-one will receive an effective service. On the other hand it may be necessary to demonstrate to colleagues in medical and surgical specialities that psychiatry has something to offer to their elderly patients, in order to gain their support in developing services. This will not be possible unless some effective service can be provided.

9.   "Clear criteria for division of responsibility must be known and accepted both inside and outside the specialties ... not influenced by lack of resources."

In the absence of a psychiatric bed a mentally ill person (with a coincidental physical illness) does not automatically become appropriate for medical admission. If resources for one speciality are grossly inadequate, there might be pressures towards this attempted solution. If geriatrician and psychiatrist see provision of a unified service as a joint responsibility, together they will attempt to negotiate other ways of dealing with the problem.

10. "Both physicians and psychiatrists should be able to make diagnoses of delirium and dementia, assess their severity and carry out appropriate investigations ..."

The presence of dementia does not in itself move the afflicted patient from the medical/ surgical domain into that of psychiatry. Each speciality may, however, need to call on the other in some circumstances in order to carry out a complete assessment, depending on the constellation of problems presented by the individual patient.

11. "The presence or absence 'of major behavioural problems ... rather than mobility should be the principal criterion for psychiatric intervention and management after initial assessment ..."

The previous guidelines (Standing Joint Committee of the British Geriatric Society and the Royal College of Psychiatrists, 1979) stressed the importance of mobility in determining the appropriate speciality to care for demented people. Mobile people with dementia were seen as more appropriate for psychiatric care and immobile people for geriatric medical care. The most recent guidelines introduce the criterion of major behavioural problems as indicating the need for psychiatric management, and this has become widely used in practice. Behavioural disturbance is difficult to manage on a ward of physically ill people, and there needs to be the capability for a rapid psychiatric response where necessary. Staff on the old age psychiatry ward are likely to have more training and experience in managing serious behavioural problems.

12. "... collaboration should involve not only physicians and psychiatrists, but also other members of the multi-disciplinary team."

This is an important aspect of liaison services. People may need care on medical wards, despite psychiatric illness. The medical nurses might value, and the patient benefit from, involvement of psychiatric nursing staff in specific circumstances, for example when the patient is acutely distressed or actively hallucinating. Similarly there may be specific circumstances where other members of the psychiatric multidisciplinary team, such as occupational therapists or clinical psychologists, might offer advice or inter-vention to their colleagues in other departments.

We have brought patients referred from the medical wards across to our day hospital for multidisciplinary assessment, but this has disadvantages as the geriatric medical staff tend not to be involved in the assessment and may then not accept the team's assessment and advice. It is easier to reach a consensus between medical and psychiatric staff if both teams are involved in a joint assessment, although this is more difficult to arrange in practice. If the person's key medical nurse is involved throughout a psychiatric assessment in the psychiatric day hospital (or the key psychiatric nurse throughout a medical assessment), it may be possible to avoid difficulties in communication and conflict of opinions.

13.   "Joint assessment depends more on the good will and cooperation of professional colleagues ... However separate assessment units should be reasonably accessible, preferably both on the ... [same] site."

Pitt & Silver (1982) described a joint unit for medically and mentally ill old people, which was thought to reduce duplication of work by both specialities and to facilitate focusing of each specialist's expertise. It was not widely copied, and it is more usual for geriatricians and psychiatrists to have separate facilities. The well-known Department of Health Care of the Elderly in Nottingham (Arie & Jolley, 1982) maintains separate services which are run jointly in close proximity. The most important factors in joint working are probably trust and a shared philosophy of caring for older people, but in practice these can lead to different working models.

14.   "Reciprocal training ... should be mandatory ..."

Reciprocal training was one of the recommendations of the joint report of the Royal Colleges of Physicians and Psychiatrists (1989). In old age psychiatry the arrangement is flexible at present, although senior registrars in the speciality are encouraged, where appropriate, to study for the Diploma in Geriatric Medicine (DGM). Some trainees may have already obtained post-registration medical experience before entering psychiatry and feel that this is sufficient for their training in old age psychiatry; others find that this is a stimulus to further study for the DGM. Others have limited training experience in medical problems in late life: studying for the DGM may help to make up this deficit, will be appreciated by future appointments committees, and will benefit their patients. In districts where the geriatric medical service is limited, it will be an advantage for consultant old age psychiatrists to have additional medical experience. It has been claimed that physicians are more likely to respect a psychiatrist who has an additional qualification in medicine or geriatric medicine.

15. "... consultants in both [specialities] should have continuing involvement in, and influence on, ... joint planning."

This important principle will apply to planning to meet the needs of physically ill people for psychiatric care and vice versa, in addition to the other aspects of care of the elderly.

16. "The guidelines ... are as relevant to the management of patients referred from other hospital settings ..."

Although psychiatrists providing liaison services to elderly people may be able to target their service using the accumulation of older people in geriatric medical beds, they will need to take account of the many older people in other beds throughout the medical and surgical specialities of the general hospital and to work out how best to respond to their needs. It is essential for an old age psychiatrist in a large general hospital to allocate time to see patients on these wards and to liaise with the staff caring for these people.

It takes much longer to communicate well with staff if you work with them infrequently and their skills in dealing with psychiatric problems are an unknown quantity. I breathe more easily if a patient with combined physical and mental disorders is in a geriatric bed because I know what I can expect of my geriatric physician colleagues, and they know what to expect of me. They ask me questions that I can answer. On other wards, much more time is often required to talk with medical and nursing staff than to assess the patient, in order to discuss their management of the patient and the possible psychiatric contribution. Much of this work could be carried out more effectively by suitably trained old age psychiatry liaison nurses, who would have more time to develop a relationship with staff in other departments of the hospital and could also demonstrate appropriate nursing skills. The potential contribution of such nursing posts has not yet been adequately evaluated.

Conclusions

Liaison psychiatry referrals may initiate around half of the work of an old age psychiatry district service and therefore require a commensurate allocation of resources. It is essential that services are balanced between the needs of community and hospital and to recognise that there is a considerable overlap between them. Liaison services improve the quality of care and shorten hospital stays, and therefore are cost effective.

Medical and other staff sessions should be allocated for the provision of liaison psychiatry. Otherwise, elderly people with both physical and mental disorders will be disadvantaged. This is particularly likely in a setting of community-orientated care. Job plans of consultants in old age psychiatry should include sessions for liaison work, and other resources must be identified to support this service. One way of ensuring that the needs of these elderly people are provided for may be to appoint old age psychiatry liaison nurses who work only with this group of people. These nurses will be able to establish close relationships both with other departments of the hospital and with other members of the old age psychiatry team. All old age psychiatry staff who are involved in providing liaison psychiatry services require specific knowledge and skills and these must be included in their training.

Further research is needed to identify the needs of elderly patients in medical and surgical wards, the effects of treatment provided, and the extent to which these needs are met using different models of service provision. Guidelines have been agreed for planning liaison services for the elderly, and should be included in the criteria which are applied to audit services.

References

ARIE, T. & JOLLEY, D. J. (1982) Making services work: organisation and style of psychogeriatric services. In *The Psychiatry of Late Life* (eds R. Levy & F. Post). Oxford: Blackwell.

BENBOW, S. M. (1987) Liaison referrals to a department of psychiatry for the elderly 1984–5. *International Journal of Geriatric Psychiatry*, **2**, 235–240.

BROWN, L. M. & McEVOY, A. W. (1993) A joint assessment ward for the elderly. Presented at the Section of Old Age Psychiatry Conference, Royal College of Psychiatrists, Glasgow.

DOVER, S. & McWILLIAM, C. (1992) Physical illness associated with depression in the elderly in community based and hospital patients. *Psychiatric Bulletin*, **16**, 612–613.

FELDMAN, E., MAYOU, R., HAWTON, K., *et al* (1987) Psychiatric disorder in medical in-patients. *Quarterly Journal of Medicine*, **63**, 405–412.

FOLKS, D. G. & FORD, C. V. (1985) Psychiatric disorders in geriatric medical/surgical patients. Part I: report of 195 consecutive consultations. *Southern Medical Journal*, **78**, 239–241.

LEVITAN, S. J. & KORNFELD, D. S. (1981) Clinical and cost benefits of liaison psychiatry. *American Journal of Psychiatry*, **138**, 790–793.

LICHTENSTEIN, H. & WINOGRAD, C. H. (1984) Geriatric consultation: a functional approach. *Journal of the American Geriatrics Society*, **32**, 356–361.

LIPOWSKI, Z. J. (1983) The need to integrate liaison psychiatry and gero-psychiatry. *American Journal of Psychiatry*, **140**, 1003–1005.

MILLAR, H. R. (1981) Psychiatric morbidity in elderly surgical patients. *British Journal of Psychiatry*, **138**, 17–20.

MURDOCH, P. S. & MONTGOMERY, E. A. (1992) Revised guidelines for collaboration between physicians in geriatric medicine and psychiatrists of old age. *Psychiatric Bulletin*, **16**, 583–584.

MURPHY, E., SMITH, R., LINDESEY, J., *et al* (1988) Increased mortality rates in late-life depression. *British Journal of Psychiatry*, **152**, 347–353.

O'RIORDAN, T. G., HAYES, J. P., SHELLEY, R., *et al* (1989) The prevalence of depression in an acute geriatric medical assessment unit. *International Journal of Geriatric Medicine*, **4**, 17–21.

PITT, B. (1993) The liaison psychiatry of old age. In *Recent Advances in Clinical Psychiatry*, vol. 8 (ed. K. Granville–Grossman). Edinburgh: Churchill Livingstone.

—— & SILVER, C. P. (1982) The combined psychogeriatric approach. In *Medicine and Psychiatry: a Practical Approach* (eds J. M. Pfeffer & F. H. Creed). London: Pitman.

RAMSAY, R., WRIGHT, P., KATZ, A., *et al* (1991) The detection of psychiatric morbidity and its effects on outcome in acute elderly medical admissions. *International Journal of Geriatric Psychiatry*, **6**, 881–886.

ROYAL COLLEGE OF PHYSICIANS AND ROYAL COLLEGE OF PSYCHIATRISTS' JOINT WORKING PARTY (1989) *Specialist Services and Medical Training for the Care of Elderly People with Mental Illness*. London: Royal College of Psychiatrists.

ROZZINI, R., BIANCHETTI, A., CARABELLESI, C., *et al* (1988) Depression, life events and somatic symptoms. *Gerontologist*, **28**, 229–232.

SADAVOY, J., SMITH, I., CONN, D. K., *et al* (1990) Depression in geriatric patients with chronic mental illness. *International Journal of Geriatric Psychiatry*, **5**, 187–192.

SHAH, A., PHONGSATHORN, V., GEORGE, C., *et al* (1992) Psychiatric morbidity among continuing care geriatric patients. *International Journal of Geriatric Psychiatry*, **7**, 517–525.

STANDING JOINT COMMITTEE OF THE BRITISH GERIATRIC SOCIETY AND THE ROYAL COLLEGE OF PSYCHIATRISTS (1979) Guidelines for collaboration between geriatric physicians and psychiatrists in the care of the elderly. *Bulletin of the Royal College of Psychiatrists*, November, 168–169.

STRAIN, J. J., LYONS, J. S., HAMMER, J. S., *et al* (1991) Cost offset from a consultation-liaison intervention with elderly hip fracture patients. *American Journal of Psychiatry*, **148**, 1044–1049.

Part III. Education and research in liaison psychiatry

10 Undergraduate teaching

GARY BELL

The educational role of liaison psychiatry is concerned not only with increasing the ability of medical staff to detect psychiatric disorders in their patients and make appropriate referrals, but also with the development of their therapeutic skills, most notably communication skills which will be of use both in hospital medicine and in general practice. It is essential, therefore, that the teaching of liaison psychiatry is given a high profile in the undergraduate curriculum if these objectives are to be realised.

While a good grounding in basic medical sciences is the main aim of preclinical training, a common and unfortunate byproduct is a narrow biological view of disease. Teaching medical students about the contribution of life events, chronic social and interpersonal difficulties and personality factors to the aetiology, course and prognosis of an individual patient's illness helps to redress this imbalance. Students also need to learn the value of developing a relationship with the patient and the importance of exploring the patient's view of his or her illness.

The setting

It is inevitable that the opportunities to expose medical students to liaison work during their psychiatry clerkship will vary greatly, even within the same medical school. The bulk of liaison psychiatry teaching, therefore, should take place on general medical firms in both the first and third clinical years of the curriculum: that is, both before and after the psychiatry clerkship. Teaching sessions should occur once a week throughout the medical clerkships (usually 8 to 12 weeks), preferably on the medical ward where the student is currently working and involving an interview with a patient. The first session should be used to outline the aims and objectives of the teaching sessions and, wherever possible, include a brief presentation of, and an interview with, a patient recently seen in the course of the psychiatrist's routine liaison work.

The content

First clinical year

The emphasis in the first clinical year should be on developing interview skills, the importance of the doctor–patient relationship and the relevance of psychosocial factors to the patient's physical illness. Students should therefore be encouraged to select patients with seemingly uncomplicated physical illnesses for the weekly teaching sessions. The selection of suitable patients for such teaching sessions should be made by the liaison psychiatrist in consultation with the medical registrar on the students' firm.

Important areas to explore are the patients' reactions to their illness and hospitalisation, the extent to which they feel able to discuss matters with their doctors, and their concerns for the future. Interviewing the patient after the student's presentation is an excellent opportunity to demonstrate good interview skills. Students also have the opportunity to discover how grateful many patients are for the opportunity to discuss a number of concerns such as sexual problems and the fear of dying – subjects about which many students feel awkward, and yet when discussed, are often of great relief to the patients.

Occasionally there will be patients with typical somatising disorders, including hysteria, in whom it is possible to demonstrate in a very dramatic and convincing way the relationship of psycho-logical and social factors to physical symptoms. However, such patients should not dominate teaching sessions at the expense of those with common physical disorders such as myocardial infarction, stroke, and chronic respiratory and gastrointestinal disorders.

Third clinical year

Invariably there will be considerable overlap in the types of patient used in the teaching of liaison psychiatry to first and third year medical students. Teaching of third year students provides the opportunity to incorporate the skills of assessment, diagnosis and management of psychiatric disorders learnt during the psychiatry clerkship. This allows students to see the relevance of such skills in settings other than an acute psychiatric admission ward or an out-patient clinic. Students should be given the opportunity to present patients with acute and chronic organic brain disorders, problems of drug and alcohol misuse, atypical or unexplained somatic disorders, poor compliance, eating disorders and deliberate self-harm. The use of appropriate out-patients will help ensure that as wide a variety of patients and conditions as possible are seen. This is especially important given the increasingly short period of in-patient stays, and the trend towards out-patient treatment of many conditions.

Getting the balance right is important. The students should develop a truly integrated approach to the assessment, diagnosis and management of their patients' illnesses, but the automatic assumption that unexplained physical symptoms have a psychosocial origin is to be discouraged.

It is well established that a great deal of minor to moderate psychiatric morbidity, in particular anxiety and depression, goes undetected by medical staff on general medical wards. The use of the General Health Questionnaire (28-item version) by medical students in a general medical setting has been shown to be useful in increasing factual knowledge about otherwise undetected psychiatric morbidity, and in improving skills at identifying and treating such illnesses (McGrath *et al*, 1986). The incorporation of a few carefully selected questions, designed to detect psychiatric morbidity, into standard medical clerking may well prove a useful adjunct to liaison teaching sessions.

Assessment and feedback

The students

What should students learn from liaison teaching sessions? Assessment of communication skills and attitudes to patients is far more difficult than assessment of the factual knowledge gained. Despite this, it is essential that this is done if liaison teaching is to make inroads into other areas of the clinical course, for example, surgery, obstetrics, paediatrics and geriatrics. Every academic department of psychiatry should establish regular assessment of student feedback in order to argue for curriculum time and resources.

responsibility for them between the physician or casualty consultant and the psychiatrist. A few training centres provide more extensive experience of the use of liaison psychiatry beds (see Chapter 6). The consultant in liaison psychiatry will inevitably have responsibility for coordinating the service for self-poisoning in the general hospital. It is imperative that the trainee should have a good grasp of this subject, personal experience of assessing many patients who have taken an overdose, and involvement in organising the service.

As the trainee gains experience, he/she should have increasing opportunities to teach and supervise more junior trainees, and in teaching hospitals should be involved in teaching medical students on the medical and surgical wards. It is mandatory that all aspects of this work are supervised by a consultant who has a particular commitment to liaison psychiatry.

Undertaking clinical research

It is important that the liaison psychiatrist has some experience of research for two main reasons. Firstly, research in the relatively new field of liaison psychiatry is burgeoning and there are likely to be further developments (see Chapter 12). In order to appraise new research and understand the instruments that are being used to assess patients, one should have had research experience oneself. Secondly, one of the best ways of forging links with the general hospital is through the development of joint research projects. This leads to a better and closer relationship with the physician or surgeon and generates additional referrals.

Gaining management experience

This should include the management experience required to be a general psychiatrist, and involve the attendance of management courses and a familiarity with the current changes in health service administration.

In addition, the trainee should have experience of applying clinical audit in the liaison setting. As managerial skills will be important for consultants in the future, the trainee may consider 'shadowing' a consultant in liaison psychiatry, in regard to his/her managerial commitments, for a few months. This will involve attending policy meetings, reading documents and being involved in the development of services. Planning documents of many hospitals often omit the provision of psychiatric care for hospital in-patients. It will be essential for the future development of liaison psychiatry that psychiatrists are able to argue cogently and forcefully for the maintenance or expansion of a service, and that they can skilfully negotiate and barter with other medical colleagues and managers.

Specific recommendations

Based on these general principles, the Executive Committee of the Liaison Psychiatry Group of the Royal College has produced recommendations for minimum training requirements in liaison psychiatry – both at SHO/registrar and senior registrar level (House & Creed, 1993). These (adapted) recommendations are set out in the Appendix.

References

HOUSE, A. & CREED, F. (1993) Training in liaison psychiatry: recommendations from the Liaison Psychiatry Group Executive Committee. *Psychiatric Bulletin*, **17**, 95–96.

MAYOU, R., ANDERSON, H., FEINMANN, C., *et al* (1990) The present state of consultation and liaison psychiatry. *Psychiatric Bulletin*, **14**, 321–325.

12   The relevance of research

ELSPETH GUTHRIE and FRANCIS CREED

Recent years have seen increasing interest in research in liaison psychiatry. However, the field is still relatively new and knowledge remains limited in many areas. The development of high quality consultation–liaison services will depend upon detailed knowledge of the nature and extent of psychological morbidity in the general hospital, and also upon an understanding of the needs of physicians and non-medical personnel involved in the care of patients with psychiatric disorder. In addition, careful evaluation of the effectiveness of psychiatric intervention in different disorders needs to be undertaken, highlighting the special skills required to treat some patients. A brief summary follows of the particular areas of liaison psychiatry that have been adequately researched. Areas that require further detailed investigation, which should become the focus of research in the foreseeable future, will be indicated.

Prevalence of psychiatric morbidity

Both in-patients and out-patients at the general hospital have higher levels of psychiatric morbidity than the general population. The prevalence of psychiatric disorder in the hospital setting varies from 13–61% for in-patients to 14–52% for out-patients (Mayou & Hawton, 1986). About a quarter of all patients on general medical wards (excluding those admitted for self-harm) have some form of psychiatric disorder (Maguire *et al*, 1974), with affective disorders and acute organic problems being the most common. Alcohol problems are found in 18% of men and 4% of women admitted to general medical wards (Feldman *et al*, 1987).

The range of prevalence figures quoted by different studies reflects the different populations of patients under investigation and the different methodologies and measures employed. Individuals with functional or non-organic symptoms have a higher prevalence of psychiatric disorder than those with organic disease. For example, patients attending a gastroenterology department with functional bowel disorder have significantly higher rates of psychiatric disorder than those with organic bowel disease (Creed & Guthrie, 1987).

The method of assessment of psychological disorder needs to be noted. Assessments based on clinical judgement (Gomez & Dally, 1977) yield very high rates of psychiatric morbidity and should always be treated with extreme caution. Clinical interviews are the best way of assessing patients with physical illness, as they have the capacity to exclude somatic symptoms resulting from physical illness, which may otherwise be attributed to a psychological cause. Self-report questionnaires may be unable to do this and can result in inflated estimates of psychological morbidity.

Types of disorders

As consultation–liaison services have developed, there has been increasing concern that the standard classification systems used in general psychiatry are inadequate to categorise patients referred to psychiatrists within the general hospital. The main problem is the coexistence of physical illness and its complex interaction with psychiatric disorder and personality. Thomas (1983) developed a new system and classified patients according to type of clinical problem rather than diagnosis. He described seven main categories: psychological reaction to illness; somatic presentation of psychiatric disorder; coincidental psychiatric disorder; cerebral complications of physical illness; abnormal behaviour causing physical illness; psychosomatic disorder; and no psychiatric disorder.

The two most common categories were 'somatic presentation of psychiatric disorder' and 'psychological reaction to physical illness'. Examples of patients fitting these two categories would be, in the first , a patient who presented with weight loss and low appetite who was suffering from a depressive illness, and, in the second, a patient with breast cancer who subsequently became depressed. Many patients who present with somatic symptoms for which no underlying organic cause can be found, and in which psychological factors seem to be important, are also included in the first category.

Needs of physicians

The needs of physicians and other non-medical staff with regard to consultation–liaison services have not been fully established, but many physicians would like closer collaboration with psychiatrists. Nearly all the physicians surveyed in Oxford by Mayou & Smith (1986) considered management of emotional problems as an important part of their clinical work and expressed the wish to do more of it themselves. They also looked to psychiatrists for more help; 61% requested better educational aids and 68% wanted more contact with the psychiatric service. Many suggested joint meetings.

Part of the role of the liaison psychiatrist needs to be in educating other hospital staff so that they can identify patients with psychiatric illness. Not all patients with psychiatric disorder need to see a psychiatrist but, as consultation–liaison services develop, the two most common types of problem ('somatic presentation of psychiatric disorder' and 'psychological reaction to physical illness') are referred at an increased rate (Sensky *et al*, 1985). This suggests that not only are these the two most common types of psychological problem in the general hospital, but they are also the ones with which physicians require most help.

Creed *et al* (1993) suggest that as a good consultation–liaison service develops, physicians and surgeons begin to identify and refer patients who previously would not have received psychiatric help. In addition, their study shows that up to half of all referrals to a liaison psychiatrist can be adequately managed by the referring doctor, with advice from the psychiatrist. In the vast majority of referrals to a liaison service, the referring doctor requests advice regarding either diagnosis or treatment (Creed *et al*, 1993). It is rare for the psychiatrist to be asked to take over completely the management of the patient, although it is not unknown for some psychiatrists to behave in a defensive and unhelpful way, because they assume that this is what the referring doctor wants.

Referral and treatment

Consultation–liaison services in the UK have been primarily concerned with the assessment of self-poisoning patients (Mayou & Lloyd, 1985). For other clinical problems there is a huge discrepancy between the prevalence of psychiatric disorders in medical in-patients (approximately 20%) and the actual referral rate to psychiatrists (less than 1%) (Mayou, 1989). Low priority has been given to developing liaison services in district planning

(Kingdon, 1989) and general psychiatrists have not encouraged referrals from the general hospital for fear of the "floodgates opening". As a new liaison service develops, it receives an increased number of referrals, and it is important to recognise that a good quality service cannot be attained without the availability of additional resources.

Studies of treatment in liaison psychiatry have been patchy and very variable in quality. It is a huge area, encompassing many different physical conditions and a wide variety of psychological problems. There have been relatively few studies of the overall impact of the introduction of a liaison service to a general medical setting. In a controlled trial, Gater *et al* (1994) found that psychiatric intervention made little difference to the overall long-term psychiatric morbidity of patients, although the cost of treatment in terms of subsequent readmissions was reduced. This is in marked contrast to other work (Strain *et al*, 1991) which targeted a particular group of patients – elderly people with hip fractures – and demonstrated that routine psychiatric intervention resulted in early detection of psychiatric morbidity, better psychiatric care, earlier discharge and substantial cost savings for the hospital. When interpreting the results of these two papers, it is important to bear in mind the differing groups of patients studied. In the first study, many of the patients were seriously ill with chronic conditions and in fact later died, whereas in the second study the patients had an acute condition that could be treated in a straightforward manner and were generally in better physical health.

These two studies highlight the difficulties of making comparisons and drawing conclusions regarding treatment effect in the field of liaison psychiatry. Most treatment interventions employed in liaison psychiatry are similar to those in the rest of psychiatry and include: drugs, psychotherapy, cognitive therapy and behavioural techniques. There are many case reports and descriptions of particular psychological interventions, but few methodologically sound controlled treatment trials.

The identification of psychological sequelae of cancer, and the development of various treatment approaches including counselling, drug treatment (Maguire *et al*, 1980) and cognitive therapy (Greer, 1985) have made an enormous impact and have acted as models for the development of treatment interventions in other physical conditions.

A growing awareness of the cost involved to the National Health Service of treating patients with somatising disorders has led to increased interest in developing psychological strategies to help these patients. Svedlund (1983) and Guthrie *et al* (1991) have demonstrated the beneficial effects of brief dynamic therapy in the majority of patients with chronic irritable bowel syndrome, and Klimes *et al* (1990) have shown that brief cognitive–behavioural therapy can alleviate physical symptoms in patients with atypical noncardiac chest pain.

Patients with somatisation can be represented on a continuum. At one end are individuals who are aware that their physical symptoms have a psychological aetiology and are responsive to psychological intervention. These individuals are disproportionately represented in new referrals with non-organic disease at medical out-patient clinics. At the other end of the spectrum are patients with somatisation who firmly believe that their symptoms have a physical aetiology, are resistant to any psychological intervention, and who continue to seek medical care, often utilising a great deal of Health Service resources. These patients account for a sizeable proportion of the re-attenders with non-organic disease at medical out-patient clinics.

It may be premature to assess the overall impact of these studies on the practice of liaison psychiatry, but they have raised several important issues. Firstly, patients with relatively mild somatisation may respond to fairly simple psychological interventions, if they are treated at or near the point of referral. Patients who are chronic attenders are less amenable to psychiatric intervention, and require more intensive treatments from skilled therapists (see Chapter 2). Some patients with severe somatisation are unlikely to respond to out-patient treatment. These are best managed by either offering in-patient behavioural treatment (Bass & Benjamin, 1993) or limiting further inappropriate investigations or treatment by liaising closely with the referring doctor. Finally, the role of psychotropic drugs in the treatment of somatisation disorders has yet to be clearly established.

Special skills and training

The practice of consultation–liaison psychiatry requires the acquisition and development of particular skills. In addition to detailed knowledge of the psychiatric and psychological sequelae of physical illness, the psychiatrist needs to be able to interview and engage somatising patients in treatment. Recent workshops organised by the Liaison Psychiatry Group of the Royal College of Psychiatrists have resulted in the documentation of the various approaches and techniques required for interviewing somatising patients (Creed & Guthrie, 1993) and the methods employed for their treatment (Bass & Benjamin, 1993). Gask *et al* (1989) focused on whether it is possible to teach doctors to interview these patients more skilfully, and whether doctors can also be taught specific psychological techniques to help somatising patients to make a link between their physical symptoms and psychological status.

Areas for future research

Relatively few areas of liaison psychiatry have been adequately researched to date. The two areas that have received most attention have been: (a) the assessment of overt psychological morbidity (such as anxiety and depression) amongst general hospital patients; and (b) the recognition of the high prevalence of non-organic physical complaints in medical out-patients. There are some specialities like neurology and gastroenterology where numerous reports and studies of the prevalence of psychiatric disorder repeat work that has already been done, and so do not add to the overall body of knowledge. On the other hand there are specialities such as oral surgery where the level of psychological morbidity is just beginning to be identified, and further investigation is required.

The four areas of liaison psychiatry in most need of further development and research in the near future are as follows:

The cost of unnecessary physical investigations

The mechanisms available in this country for accurately quantifying the cost of medical treatment and investigation are still very crude. Admissions for 'non-specific abdominal pain' alone have been estimated to cost £16.5 million a year in the UK (Raheja *et al*, 1990). It is likely that simple forms of psychiatric intervention may help to reduce such costs provided specific conditions are targeted. There is an urgent need for methodologically sound research that can accurately assess the cost of certain medical conditions and demonstrate the savings that would be made by appropriate psychiatric treatment.

Development of new psychological treatment strategies

Some psychiatric conditions in the general hospital setting are relatively straightforward to treat, such as a depressive illness in a patient following multiple fractures incurred in a road traffic accident. Some other conditions, such as the treatment of a patient with a depressive illness who is unable to tolerate anti-depressant medication because of his renal failure, may be more complicated. For conditions such as the somatoform disorders, appropriate and effective forms of treatment are still being developed. Further research comparing the effectiveness of different interventions in conditions such as chronic fatigue syndrome is required. From a practical perspective, research that enables clinicians to identify more easily those patients with somatising disorders that will respond successfully to brief psychiatric interventions will be very helpful.

Closer liaison with medical staff

Not all patients with psychiatric disorder in the general hospital need to be seen by a psychiatrist. Medical staff, however, require guidance and training from psychiatrists in order to deal with patients' psychological problems more easily. Although work has been carried out in general practice, very little research has been conducted into whether physicians can be taught to interview more empathically and manage patients' psychological distress in a helpful way. Changing the behaviour of physicians could help to reduce the cost of hospital investigations and treatment.

Many psychiatrists run liaison psychiatry services in a similar fashion to the way in which some community psychiatric clinics are conducted in general practice. These so-called 'shifted out-patient clinics' often result in very little liaison or discussion with GPs, a relatively small number of patients are seen, and GPs are not helped to improve and develop their psychiatric skills. This style of working is often repeated by liaison psychiatrists in general hospitals. Further research needs to be carried out into more imaginative and flexible styles of service delivery. The effect of psychiatrists adapting their mode of working to place more emphasis on discussion with physicians and surgeons needs to be evaluated.

The A&E department and management of deliberate self-harm

The accident and emergency (A&E) department requires special mention. It is a new speciality with many aspects of service that are relevant to liaison psychiatry. For example, recent research (Mayou, 1992) suggests that the psychological and social causes and consequences of road traffic accidents deserve greater attention. Psychiatric consequences are common and include post-traumatic stress disorder and phobic travel anxiety.

The management and prevention of deliberate self-harm accounts for a large proportion of the work carried out by the A&E department. Research into this area has been given added impetus by the priorities outlined in the Department of Health's recent *Health of the Nation* document (National Health Service Management Executive, 1993).

Future directions for liaison psychiatry

Liaison psychiatry as a speciality is now at a critical developmental point. Although centres of excellence have been established in the UK (Anderson, 1989; Mayou *et al*, 1990), these have mainly been in teaching hospitals. A lack of time and resources has prevented psychiatrists in district general hospitals from providing anything other than a skeleton liaison service (Mayou *et al*, 1990). If the psychological welfare of medical patients is to be improved, additional resources will be required. Funds from the mental illness budget should be sought for a well organised and closely supervised deliberate self-harm service. Funding from medical and surgical units will be required for additional psychiatric sessions for general hospital patients. The success of the latter will depend upon the quality of the collaboration which is now developing between physicians, surgeons and psychiatrists.

The liaison psychiatrist needs to be at the forefront of changing attitudes towards psychiatry in the general hospital. Appropriate psychological care of general medical patients, including psychiatric referral where appropriate, should become accepted as a measurable aspect of quality in the general hospital. Once referral has occurred, the liaison psychiatrist must respond positively. Where appropriate, the patient must be actively engaged, a diagnosis made, and a clear treatment and management plan worked out. Better use of and collaboration with non-medical staff, who may not be funded from the mental health budget, should occur (Maguire & Sellwood, 1982; Rumsey, 1991). In addition, careful audit measures should be employed to evaluate critically the effectiveness of the liaison service.

Creed (1992) has suggested that one invaluable result of research in liaison psychiatry will be the development of agreed algorithms for specific problems. These will act as a guide to help reduce the cost of unnecessary investigation and improve patient care. For example, at the initial assessment of a patient with functional abdominal pain, both physical and psychological aspects of the patient need to be addressed. A certain number of physical investigations may be regarded as reasonable to exclude organic disease, as should the inclusion of a number of questions regarding psychological and social issues. The explanation given to the patient of the resulting findings should be positive, clear and compatible with the patient's previous ideas and beliefs. Such a schema could be readily followed, and is easy to audit.

Different algorithms would have to be worked out for difficult conditions and situations. The requirements of a patient with chest pain may be different from those of a patient with abdominal pain. It may be possible, however, to develop gradually a whole series of different schema to help physicians improve psychological management. The design of such approaches, and the evaluation of their efficacy, will be important goals for future research.

This kind of collaborative endeavour will require psychiatrists to take time, with their physician colleagues, to work out appropriate guidelines. Such a close working relationship is a hallmark of good liaison psychiatry and will not only benefit patients but may lead to new, previously unexplored, avenues of research.

Conclusions

Liaison psychiatry is a rapidly growing speciality. Research in this field has developed particularly in the last 15 years. In this short space of time, the high level of psychiatric morbidity in hospital in-patients and out-patients has been clearly established and the most common kinds of psychiatric disorder that occur in the hospital setting have been identified. The search for the most appropriate psychiatric interventions for these different conditions has begun, and the efficacy of psychological treatment for some conditions has already been established. The psychiatrist's style and mode of practice needs to change with the aim of developing closer colla-boration with medical and surgical departments. It is a huge field with wide ranging possibilities for further research. Better classification systems and further controlled treatment studies are essential, and more detailed study of the complex interaction between physical and psychological processes is required.

References

ANDERSON, H. M. (1989) Liaison psychiatry in Scotland: the present service. *Psychiatric Bulletin,* **13,** 606–608.

BASS, C. & BENJAMIN, S. (1993) Management of chronic somatisation. *British Journal of Psychiatry,* **162,** 472–480.

CREED, F. H. (1992) The future of liaison psychiatry in the UK. *International Review of Psychiatry,* **4,** 99–107.

—— & GUTHRIE, E. (1987) Psychological factors in the irritable bowel syndrome. *Gut,* **28,** 1307–1318.

—— & —— (1993) Techniques for interviewing the somatising patient. *British Journal of Psychiatry,* **162,** 467–471.

——, ——, BLACK, D., *et al* (1993) Psychiatric referrals within the general hospital-comparison with GP referrals. *British Journal of Psychiatry,* **162,** 204–211.

FELDMAN, E., MAYOU, R., HAWTON, K., *et al* (1987) Psychiatric disorder in medical in-patients. *Quarterly Journal of Medicine, New Series,* **63,** 405–412.

GASK, L., GOLDBERG, D. & PORTER, R. (1989) The treatment of somatization: evaluation of a teaching package with general practice trainees. *Journal of Psychosomatic Research*, **33**, 697–703.

GATER, R., GOLDBERG, D., EVANSON, J., *et al* (1993) The detection and treatment of psychiatric illness in a general medical ward: a cost–utility analysis. *Journal of Psychosomatic Research* (in press).

GOMEZ, J. & DALLY, P. (1977) Psychologically mediated abdominal pain in surgical and medical out-patient clinics. *British Medical Journal*, **I**, 1451–1453.

GREER, S. (1985) Cancer: psychiatric aspects. In *Recent Advances in Clinical Psychiatry* (ed. W. Granville-Grossman). Edinburgh: Churchill Livingstone.

GUTHRIE, E., CREED, F. H., DAWSON, D., *et al* (1991) A controlled trial of psychological treatment in the irritable bowel syndrome. *Gastroenterology*, **100**, 450–457.

KINGDON, D. (1989) Mental health services: results of a survey of English district plans. *Psychiatric Bulletin*, **13**, 77–78.

KLIMES, I., MAYOU, R. A., PEARCE, M. J., *et al* (1990) Psychological treatment for atypical non-cardiac chest pain: a controlled evaluation. *Psychological Medicine*, **20**, 605–611.

MAGUIRE, G. P., JULIER, D. L., HAWTON, K. E., *et al* (1974) Psychiatric morbidity and referral on two general medical wards. *British Medical Journal*, **I**, 268–270.

——, TAIT, A., BROOKE, M., *et al* (1980) Effect of counselling on the psychiatric morbidity associated with mastectomy. *British Medical Journal*, **I**, 1454–1456.

—— & SELLWOOD, R. (1982) A liaison psychiatry service for mastectomy patients. In *Medicine and Psychiatry: A Practical Approach* (eds F. H. Creed & J. M. Pfeffer), pp. 377–395. London: Pitman.

MAYOU, R. A. (1989) Consultation–liaison psychiatry: an international perspective. *Psychiatry Clinical Update*. Crawley: Upjohn.

—— (1992) Psychiatric aspects of road traffic accidents. *International Review of Psychiatry*, **4**, 45–54.

—— & LLOYD, G. (1985) A survey of liaison psychiatry in the United Kingdom and Eire. *Bulletin of the Royal College of Psychiatrists*, **9**, 214–217.

—— & HAWTON, K. E. (1986) Psychiatric disorder in the general hospital. *British Journal of Psychiatry*, **149**, 172–190.

—— & SMITH, E. B. O. (1986) Hospital doctors' management of psychological problems. *British Journal of Psychiatry*, **148**, 194–197.

——, ANDERSON, H., FEINMAN, C., *et al* (1990) The present state of consultation and liaison psychiatry. *Psychiatric Bulletin*, **14**, 321–325.

NATIONAL HEALTH SERVICE MANAGEMENT EXECUTIVE (1993) *Health of the Nation Key Area Handbook: Mental Illness*. London: National Health Service Management Executive.

OWENS, D., DENNIS, M., JONES, S., *et al* (1991) Self-poisoning patients discharged from accident and emergency: risk factors and outcome. *Journal of the Royal College of Physicians*, **25**, 218–222.

RAHEJA, S. K., MCDONALD, P. J. & TAYLOR, I. (1990) Non-specific abdominal pain – an expensive mystery. *Journal of Royal Society of Medicine*, **83**, 10–11.

RUMSEY, N. (1991) Groups stress management versus pharmacological treatment in the irritable bowel syndrome. In *Towards Confident Management of Irritable Bowel Syndrome* (eds K. W. Heaton, F. H. Creed & N. Goeting). Duphar Medical Relations.

SENSKY, T., GREER, S., CUNDY, T., *et al* (1985) Referrals to psychiatrists in a general hospital – comparison of two methods of liaison psychiatry: preliminary communication. *Journal of Royal Society of Medicine*, **78**, 463–468.

STRAIN, J. J., LYONS, J. S., HAMMER, J. S., *et al* (1991) Cost offset from a psychiatric consultation–liaison intervention with elderly hip fracture patients. *American Journal of Psychiatry*, **148**, 1044–1049.

SVEDLUND, J. (1983) Psychotherapy in irritable bowel syndrome: a controlled outcome study. *Acta Psychiatrica Scandinavica*, **67** (suppl. 306), 1–86.

THOMAS, C. (1983) Referrals to a British liaison psychiatry service. *Health Trends*, **15**, 61–64.

Appendix
Recommendations of the Liaison Psychiatry Group Executive Committee for postgraduate training

It is generally agreed that training in liaison psychiatry should be available at SHO/registrar grade, but the Royal College of Psychiatrists' guidelines are not specific about what it might entail. As a result it is difficult for approval visitors to decide whether a particular post on a rotational training scheme truly provides liaison experience. At times so-called 'liaison experience' amounts to no more than participation in a duty-rota for visiting a general hospital to undertake the assessment of cases of deliberate self-harm.

Senior registrars need guidance on what constitutes adequate training for a post at consultant level with an interest in (and sessional commitment to) liaison work. By the same token, appointments advisory committees need to know what criteria to apply when assessing the training of a candidate who is applying for such a post.

The Executive Committee of the Liaison Psychiatry Group believes that the College's guidelines on training at SHO/registrar grade, and the guidelines of the Joint Committee on Higher Psychiatric Training on training at senior registrar grade, should be more specific than they are. The group has agreed criteria for training in liaison psychiatry, and they are outlined here. We are aware that many schemes do not (and could not in the short-term) offer placements which meet these criteria. Nevertheless, it is our view that they are the minimum which need to be satisfied before a post is accepted as providing liaison psychiatry training.

Training at SHO/registrar grade

Identified liaison psychiatry placements

Every training scheme should offer at least one six-month placement during which the trainee obtains experience in liaison psychiatry

This Appendix is adapted from House, A. & Creed, F. (1993) Training in liaison psychiatry: recommendations from the Liaison Psychiatry Group Executive Committee. *Psychiatric Bulletin*, **17**, 95–96.

work with adults (16–65 yrs). Similar placements may also be available as part of training in old-age psychiatry but cannot substitute for experience with younger adults. It would be desirable for the liaison experience to be provided during a full-time specialist placement; a minimum of four sessions per week liaison experience during a placement with mixed responsibilities would be acceptable. Clinical liaison experience requires contact with the general hospital as part of the trainees' daily activities, and not just visiting the hospital *ad hoc.*

Defined liaison psychiatry experience

The clinical experience obtained should include work in all of the following areas:

(a) assessment of cases of deliberate self-harm
(b) assessment and management of patients referred from (and seen in) a medical setting, with:
  (i) coexistent psychopathology and physical illness
  (ii) problems of adjustment to chronic illness
  (iii) unexplained physical symptoms and other forms of somatisation
  (iv) disorders of the nervous system or other disorders leading to transient or permanent cerebral dysfunction
(c) assessment of acute psychiatric cases, use of the Mental Health Act, and crisis management in the A&E department and elsewhere in the general hospital.

Identified clinical supervision

The trainee's clinical work in liaison psychiatry should be under-taken with adequate supervision, which has the following characteristics:

(a) It is undertaken by a designated supervisor (not simply the duty psychiatrist of the day) who is a consultant with a special commitment to liaison psychiatry.
(b) There is a regularly timetabled face-to-face supervision session with the designated consultant. In addition there should be supervision of cases at the time they are seen, which must be readily available on request.
(c) There is a component of clinical teaching in the timetabled supervision. Such teaching should include theoretical and practical aspects of psychosomatic medicine and liaison psychiatry, relevant to the cases seen in the general hospital.

Training at senior registrar grade

Ideally the trainee should have had clinical experience in liaison psychiatry at SHO/registrar level of the sort outlined above. Where such experience has not been obtained at SHO/registrar grade, it should be obtained at senior registrar level under appropriate supervision.

In addition, the following types of experience should be included in a senior registrar training placement.

Clinical

    (a) Supervision by a named individual consultant with a special responsibility for providing the liaison service.
    (b) Close liaison links should be established with at least one clinical department during the attachment.
    (c) Out-patient work should be undertaken in a specialist liaison clinic held on the general hospital site.
    (d) The opportunity should be available to supervise other professionals who are undertaking liaison work.

Education

    (a) Participation in and attendance at case presentations and other joint teaching meetings held in other clinical departments.
    (b) Experience in teaching medical staff such as house physicians and A&E staff.
    (c) It is desirable for the senior registrar to have the opportunity to undertake supervised research in an area of liaison psychiatry.

Management

    (a) Experience of coordinating the running of at least one part of the liaison service.
    (b) Experience in developing and completing at least one audit project.

The exact distribution of clinical sessions will depend on the local contract, but should amount to the equivalent of six sessions per week during a placement of at least 12 months.

Index

Compiled by JOHN GIBSON

accident and emergency department 6, 10, 110–11
administration and organisation 11
affective–cognitive symptoms 27
algorithms for specific problems 111–12
amitriptyline 32
annual referral rates from district general hospital 7 (table), 8
antidepressant medication 29
atypical non-cardiac chest pain 108

burns unit, South Gwent 54–5

cancer patients 25, 30, 66–7
  community scheme 68
  evaluation of care 69
  limited intervention scheme 67
  psychological sequelae 107
  services for 65–9
  specialist nurses 67
  treatment methods 107
  ward nurse 68
child psychiatry service 70–5
  clinical service 71
  joint clinic 73
  joint training 74
  liaison meeting 72–3
  ward liaison 74–5

Christie Hospital, Manchester 68–9
cognitive therapy 30
consultant, psychiatric 3
consultation–liaison psychiatry 47
conversion disorder 17

deliberate self-harm 5–6, 111
  South Gwent service 49–51
demands, estimating 5
demands, meeting 3–15
depression 25, 26
  amitryptyline v. cognitive behavioural therapy 32
  cognitive therapy 30
  elderly patients 76
  Endicott criteria 27 (table), 31
  failure to diagnose consequences 28 (table)
  major cardiac event predictor 29
  patient unable to take antidepressant medication 110

elderly patients 76–7
  hip fracture 107
elderly people, Central Manchester service 77–90
  benefits of service 81–2
  education/training 80–1
  geriatrician associated 80

principles 82–9
  assessed clinical needs 84
  assessment by physician/
    psychiatrist 85–6
  collaboration in multi-
    disciplinary team 87–8
  cross-reference system 85
  delirium/dementia
    diagnosis 87
  division of responsibility
    86–7
  'grey area' patients 85
  guidelines 89
  joint assessment/units 88
  joint planning 89
  major behavioural problems 87
  reciprocal training 88–9
  responsibility 84
  resources adequate 86
  right of access 84
  'unity' for consumers 83–4
  referral rate increase 77–9
  resources limitation 79
  start of service 77
Endicott criteria 27 (table), 31
estimated sessional require-ments
  11 (table)
European Consultation–Liaison
  Workgroup 52, 53 (table)
expectations of other professionals
  9

functional bowel disorders 30, 105,
  108
future directions 111–12

gastroenterology 109
General Health Questionnaire 97
GHQ 30 Questionnaire 27

'hidden population' 4
hypochondriasis 17

irritable bowel syndrome 30, 105,
  108

Leeds General Infirmary 58–63
  liaison psychiatric nursing 38–
    41
    in-patient/day-patient unit
      39–40

liaison/community nurse
    40–1
  referral numbers 62–3
  referral process 61–2
  staffing 59–61
  style of service 63–4
Leeds health services 58–9
liaison nurse/nursing 34–44
  consultation skills 36–7
  liaison skills 37
  link-nurse scheme 42
  nursing process 37–8
    orientation 37–8
    supervision 38
    termination working process
      38
  role development 42–3
Liaison Psychiatry Group 3, 5
  Executive Committee
    Recommendations 114–16
liaison team resources 8

mood disorders in the medically ill
    24–32
  detection problems 25–6
  management skills 30–1
  presentation 26–7
  prevalence 24–5
  screening techniques 26
  treatment 29–30
multiple fractures, depression
    following 110
multiple sclerosis 30

needs estimation 4
neurology 109
new psychological treatment strat-
    egies 110
'non-specific abdominal pain' cost
    109

oral surgery 109
other local psychiatric services 8–9
out-patient clinic, South Gwent 53,
    54 (table)
out-patient contacts 7

pain clinics 21
parasuicide services 6, 10
physicians' needs 106

planning a liaison service 12–15
  realistic service 13–15
  unrealistic service 12–13
postgraduate training 99–103
  acquiring clinical skills 100
  clinical research 102
  knowledge-base building 101
  management experience 102–3
  practical experience 101–2
psychiatric morbidity prevalence 104–5
psychological reaction to physical illness 105, 106

research 104–12
  accident and emergency department 119–11
  algorithms for specific problems 111–12
  cost of physical investigation 109
  deliberate self-harm 111
  future areas 109–11
  new psychological treatments 110
  physicians' needs 106
  postgraduate training 102
  prevalence of psychiatric morbidity 104–5
  referral and treatment 106–8

self-poisoning patients 106
skeleton liaison service 111
skills required 108–9
somatic presentation of psychiatric illness 105, 106
somatisation, chronic 16–22

economic isssues 21–2
nature of problem 16–17
needs estimation 17–19
needs meeting 19–21
specialist services need 20–1
somatisation disorder 17
somatoform disorders 17, 18
somatoform pain disorders 17
South Gwent service 45–57
  aims 48–9
  deliberate self-harm 49–51
  educational role 55
  medical audit 56
  out-patient clinic 53, 54 (table)
  regional burns unit 54–5
  research 55
  ward referrals 51–2
style of service provision 8–9

Thomas' classification of disorders 105
time allocation 10–11
tricyclic antidepressants 29
types of disorders 105–6

undergraduate teaching 95–8
  first clinical year 96
  medical firm 98
  third clinical year 97
University of Wales' College of Medicine, MSc in Clinical Psychiatry 55
unnecessary physical investigations 109

ward referrals 6–7, 51–2
Whittington Hospital, London 71